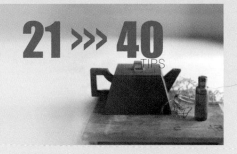
21 >>> 40 TIPS

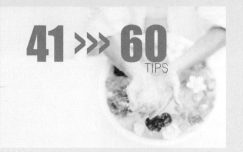
41 >>> 60 TIPS

introduction

your body overreacts

Increasing numbers of people are affected by allergies in the Western world. At least one in ten people suffers from an allergy every year. Some experience only very mild symptoms but others can become seriously ill. Allergies can sometimes even prove fatal (anaphylactic shocks or very serious asthma attacks, for example). Fortunately, such cases are relatively rare.

Although the treatment of allergies is not universally recognized as a medical discipline in the same way as, say, paediatrics or osteopathy, some doctors do specialize in it. This strange illness, which manifests itself in many forms, can affect anyone at any time, and may disappear as mysteriously as it came. It can lie dormant and then reappear years later in another form. It can even be sensitive to our moods.

tips

allergies

Marie Borrel

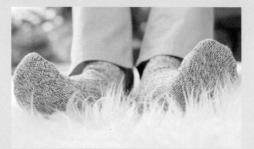

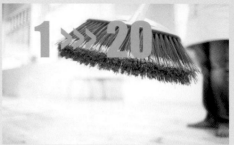

contents

introduction 4
how to use this book 7
what kind of allergy sufferer are you? 8

useful addresses 124
index 125
acknowledgements 126

Note: The information and recommendations given in this book are not intended to be a substitute for medical advice. Consult your doctor before acting on any recommendations given in this book. The authors and publisher disclaim any liability, loss, injury or damage incurred as a consequence, directly or indirectly, of the use and application of the contents of this book.

A healthy lifestyle can save us from the misery of allergies

Medical research is now taking a serious interest in the subject, and nearly three hundred new drugs to combat allergies have been patented in the last five years. Yet allergies remain stubbornly resistant to effective treatment, partly because they can be triggered by so many different factors. People suffer allergic reactions when they come into contact with allergens, and these are lurking almost everywhere in our environment. For example, the fur or saliva of pets, mould, house-dust mites in our mattresses, feathers, certain foods, pollen from flowers and trees, sunshine and sea water are all potential allergens. You are more likely to have an allergic reaction to one or several of them if your parents were sufferers. With so many potential allergens out there, both traditional and modern medicine have always had trouble finding cures for allergies, but sufferers can at least ameliorate their symptoms considerably. They can save themselves from unpleasant reactions by paying attention to what they eat, the quality of the air they breathe, the cleanliness of their homes and the cosmetics they use. A healthy lifestyle might not stop us being allergic, but it can greatly reduce the misery that allergies can cause.

Shock troops

In principle, there's nothing harmful in a cat's hair or a grain of pollen, yet they cause some people to suffer. Why? How? To answer these questions, we need to examine the very heart of our immune system. An army of microscopic soldiers is permanently on duty to defend us against attacks from germs and viruses. The immune cells meet the intruders, take note of what they are, and the next time they appear, they destroy them. This generally effective, complex and delicate system sometimes gets it wrong, however, when it mistakes a speck of dust or a harmless mite for a genuine threat and sounds the alarm. The innocent antigen (foreign body) is treated like an allergen (substance that provokes an allergic reaction).

Hardworking histamine

The immune system reacts to an intruding allergen by secreting immunoglobulins, proteins produced by white corpuscles. The immunoglobulin antibodies attach themselves to the surface of certain cells in the tissues. As soon as an allergen of the same type as the previous one appears, the immune system recognizes it and triggers a series of biological reactions, including a massive secretion of histamine. This substance, involved in all allergic reactions, spreads very quickly into the surrounding tissues. Among other things, it causes an enormous increase in the secretion of fluids and spasms in the involuntary muscles.

Histamine is responsible for the runny eyes suffered in allergic conjunctivitis, streaming noses, hay fever, the bronchial mucus characteristic of asthma, and the swollen inflammations that come with nettle rash or hives. These are just some of the consequences of the sterling efforts made by the hardworking histamine to 'protect' the body.

One mechanism, a multitude of symptoms

Just a single mechanism is able to cause a wide range of different symptoms. This is another feature peculiar to allergies: the severity of the symptoms, the form they take and the areas of the body affected differ from person to person.

An allergy should never be taken lightly, particularly if it causes violent reactions. Such cases require thorough medical treatment, but it always helps if you reinforce the treatment with a healthy lifestyle. If your reactions are not severe, a healthy lifestyle is often enough to deal with the problem. Whichever category you are in, the advice given in this book can help you.

how to use this book

> A symbol at the bottom of each page will help you to identify the natural solutions available:

Herbal medicine, aromatherapy, homeopathy, Dr Bach's flower remedies – how natural medicine can help.

Simple exercises – preventing problems by strengthening your body.

Massage and manipulation – how they help to promote well-being.

Healthy eating – all you need to know about the contribution it makes.

Practical tips for your daily life – so that you can prevent instead of having to cure.

Psychology, relaxation, Zen – advice to help you be at peace with yourself and regain serenity.

> A complete programme that will solve all your health problems.
Try it!

This book offers a made-to-measure programme, which will enable you to deal with your own particular problem. It is organized into four sections:

- **A questionnaire** to help you to assess the extent of your problem.
- **The first 20 tips** that will show you how to change your daily life in order to help prevent problems and maintain health and fitness.
- **20 slightly more radical tips** that will help you cope when problems do occur.
- **The final 20 tips** which are intended for more serious cases, when preventative measures and attempted cures have not worked.

At the end of each section someone with the same problem as you shares his or her experiences.

You can go methodically through the book from tip 1 to 60 putting each piece of advice into practice. Alternatively, you can pick out the recommendations which appear to be best suited to your particular case, or those which fit most easily into your daily routine. Or, finally, you can choose to follow the instructions according to whether you wish to prevent problems occurring or cure ones that already exist.

what kind of allergy sufferer are you?

Reply honestly to the statements below:

yes	no	1	My skin often itches.
yes	no	2	I smoke regularly.
yes	no	3	I don't pay much attention to the quality of my food.
yes	no	4	I often forget to air my home.
yes	no	5	My eyes and nose are very runny in springtime.
yes	no	6	Detergents irritate my skin.

yes	no	7	I don't do much exercise.
yes	no	8	I have a dog or cat (or several).
yes	no	9	I lose my temper very easily.

If you answered YES to statements 3, 4 and 8, Tips **1** to **20** are the ones most suited to your problems.

If you answered YES to statements 2, 5 and 7, go directly to Tips **21** to **40**.

If you answered YES to statements 1, 6 and 9, read Tips **41** to **60**.

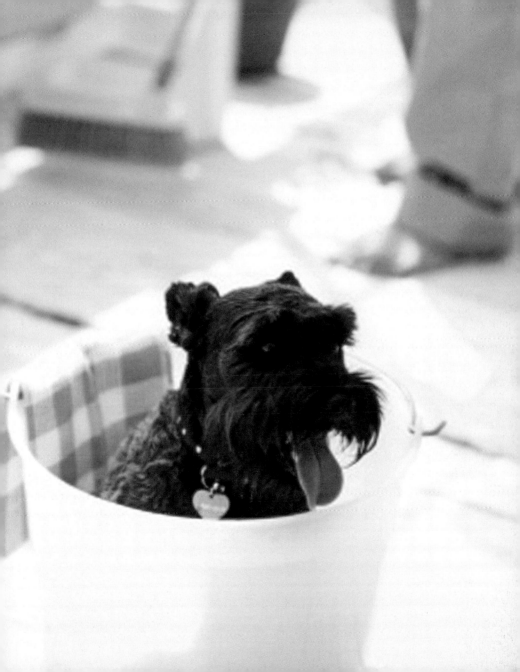

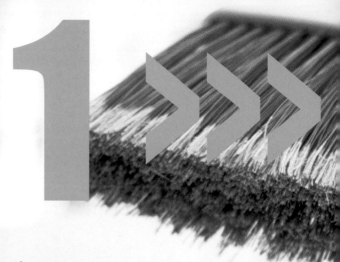

1 >>>

>> All allergies, whatever form they take, are caused by the same thing: an overreaction in your immune system. **To avoid such attacks**, you need to take some simple precautions, which can prove amazingly effective.

>>>> **First, try to discover the cause of your symptoms.** There are various ways of doing this. Then look for the culprits in your home (dust, damp or dust-mites, for instance). Keep the air clean and fresh and avoid anything that causes a reaction.

>>>>>> Avoid certain 'dangerous' foods and **eat as healthily and as naturally as possible**.

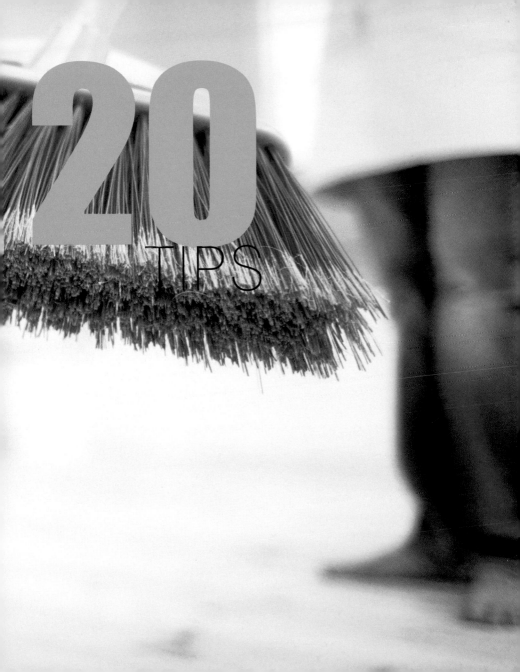

20 TIPS

01

identify your allergies

At the risk of stating the obvious, the best way of avoiding an allergic reaction is never to encounter an allergen. However, you can't begin to take the right precautions without first finding out exactly what you are allergic to.

Pollen, cat hair or strawberries?

In principle, almost anything can cause an allergy, and you need to identify your allergens in order to avoid them in the future. More often than not, people react to several substances, and it is possible to cease to be allergic to one thing only to develop an allergy to another.

Skin tests and blood tests

If you are unclear about your allergens, there are various tests to identify them.

● ● ● D I D   Y O U   K N O W ?

> These tests must be carried out or pre-scribed by a doctor, preferably a specialist in allergies. Blood tests are more reliable than skin tests, especially if the patient is allergic to more than one substance.

> When the allergen has been traced, the patient can be given desensitization treat-ment. This lasts for anything up to five years and involves introducing tiny, increasing amounts of the allergen into the body. Because of the risks of anaphylaxis, the injections have to be given in hospital, where resuscitation is available.

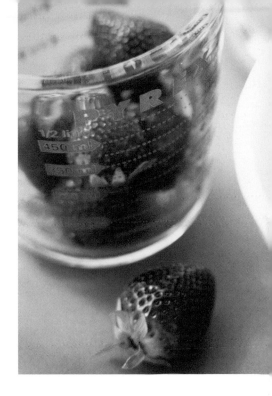

• Skin tests: the most common is the skin prick test. A drop of an allergen solution is put on the skin of the forearm and pricked into the skin with a needle. Other allergen solutions (pollen, hairs, feathers, dust, etc.) are applied, with a fresh needle each time. It only takes 10–15 minutes for any reaction to become apparent. Another skin test, the patch test, is used with patients exhibiting eczema to see if there are allergens or 'sensitizers' in creams and cosmetics. Different immune mechanisms are involved and the reaction takes 48 hours to develop. Standard batteries of allergens, together with a control, are put on the skin of the back and left in place for two or three days. A positive reaction is shown by redness and swelling.

• Blood tests: a blood sample is taken and examined for traces of specific immunoglobulins, which are antibodies produced by the immune system when an allergen is present.

> However, this treatment does not always work. And even when it does initially give good results, they are often not permanent: after a few months, or even years, the patient may become allergic to different substances.

KEY FACTS

* You can have either a blood or a skin test to help identify your allergens.

* Desensitization involves injecting gradually increasing doses of the allergen into the patient.

02

enjoy the countryside

The countryside can sometimes be terrifying for allergy sufferers, usually as a result of pollen. However, there's no need to barricade yourself inside your house because of your allergies. Just choose the right places to go and the right times to visit them.

Millions of grains of pollen

Taking exercise in the fresh air is good for you, and this applies as much to allergy sufferers as to anyone else. However, there are times when the air is filled with pollen, which invades your eyes, mouth and nose. Tree pollen appears in early spring, followed by grass pollen and the pollen of some flowers. You may well be all too familiar with what happens when you inhale it.

● ● ● DID YOU KNOW?

> Bear in mind your allergies when choosing your holiday destination. If you're allergic to iodine, take a countryside holiday instead of going to the seaside.

> If you're allergic to mites, head for the mountains: they can't survive above 1,500m (4,900ft).

Finding a solution

The air is particularly laden with pollen in the early mornings and the late afternoons, so avoid going out at these times. Rain causes pollen to fall to earth, so clearing the air. Go for a walk when it is drizzling or in the hours immediately after a heavy shower. Wear sunglasses to protect your eyes from direct contact with the pollen in the air. If you are gardening, especially mowing the lawn, wear gloves, a mask over your mouth, and glasses. Dab a little Vaseline on the edge of each nostril: it will stop a great deal of pollen from entering your airways. When you get back home, have a shower and wash your hair to remove the pollen that you've brought in with you. At the worst times of day, keep the windows closed (but see Tip 6).

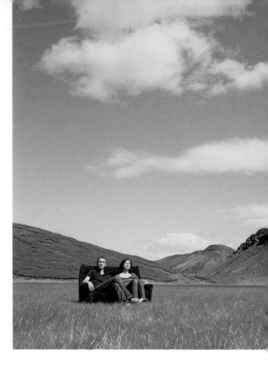

> For some countries, pollen maps are available via the Internet. They are not exact but they indicate the regions that will have high concentrations of various pollens.

KEY FACTS

* House-dust mites are so tiny they are invisible to the naked eye. They live on the flakes of skin that we shed and are found in abundance in human bedding.

* An allergen in mite faeces about the size of a pollen grain causes the problems for sufferers. The mites like warmth and damp and do badly in dry, cold air.

03

keep away from animals

Animals, including cats, dogs and horses, can adversely affect allergy sufferers. Both their hair and their saliva can trigger a reaction, as can flakes of dead skin and faeces. People with severe allergies obviously should not keep animals in the house and might need to avoid them altogether.

Cats are the worst culprits

Some people are allergic to animals and should never go near them. Cats cause the most problems: more than 40 per cent of asthma sufferers react to them. Most allergenic substances produced by cats are found in their saliva, their sebum and the fluid secreted by their eyes. These are deposited on the fur when the cat licks itself; they then dry and become airborne, which is when the

●●● DID YOU KNOW?

> An American company claims to have produced 'genetically modified cats', which have fewer allergens and don't cause allergic reactions. They will soon be available in pet stores.

> Without going to such lengths, it's useful to note that a neutered cat produces five times fewer allergens than an uncastrated one.

problems start. Dogs and horses cause fewer allergies, although their allergens are of the same kind. Reactions to birds are generally caused by mould that forms at the bottom of their cages and on their feathers.

Useful precautions

If certain animals cause you to have violent reactions, the most obvious answer is not to keep them as pets. However, if you don't want to deprive the whole household of its favourite pet, you need to take precautions.

Don't let the animal go into your bedroom and certainly don't allow it on your bed. Wash it at least once a week (this applies even to cats). Install air purifiers with fine, delicate filters to reduce the number of allergens in the air. If you keep birds or fish, always make sure that their cage or tank is scrupulously clean. In particular, stop birdcages from becoming damp. As far as possible, avoid furniture and furnishings where allergens can take up residence, such as armchairs with cloth coverings, carpets and wall-hangings. Instead, choose dry, hard coverings like parquet, vinyl and leather (for armchairs and sofas).

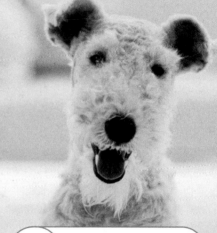

> Remember the animal does not have to be physically present to cause problems. Its shed skin and hairs cause the problems.

KEY FACTS

* Pets can cause allergic reactions.

* The simplest answer is to ban all pets from the home. If that's not possible, make sure your pet doesn't get into your bedroom.

* Wash the animal at least once a week and avoid furniture and furnishings that provide sanctuary for allergens.

04 do without flowers

Flowers might brighten up your home, but they can cause allergic reactions. If you are sensitive to flowers, you must learn to live without them.

No flowers means no pollen Cut flowers retain their pistil and stamens. As a result, they continue to spread pollen even after they have been arranged and put in a vase. If you want to keep an element of the garden inside, try non-flowering houseplants instead. These plants also have the added benefit of helping to clean the air by attracting certain harmful substances, particularly volatile organic compounds.

Choose with care If you feel you really can't do without flowers, there are certain guidelines you must follow. Firstly, make sure they are fully open. Arums and lilies, for example, have large stamens that are easy to find and remove. Wear gloves and pull out the stamens from each flower before putting them in the vase. Avoid small flowers with lots of tiny, delicate stamens. Never put flowers, or even plants, in your bedroom or your children's bedrooms.

KEY FACTS

* Cut flowers continue to spread pollen.

* Choose large flowers and remove their stamens before putting them in a vase.

05 out with insects

A bee, wasp or mosquito sting can sometimes precipitate a very dangerous allergic reaction. Beware of cockroaches, too.

As old as the pyramids Back in 3000 BC the Pharaoh Menes was killed by a wasp sting. Insect stings and food allergies (see Tips 15, 16 and 17) are the main causes of anaphylactic shock. Allergy sufferers need to be very wary of these creatures.

Reduce the risk Wasps, hornets and other flying insects all make a buzzing sound, so at least you can hear them coming and take evasive action. Cockroaches are more surreptitious. These universally loathed insects live in sinks, near drainpipes and sometimes in cupboards. Their allergens are contained in their excreta. To eradicate them, you need to locate the places they like best – warm, damp areas near to waste food – and make them spotless. Two other important points to remember: never leave dirty dishes in the sink; and store food in sealed plastic containers.

● ● ● DID YOU KNOW?

> You can also regularly use an insecticide specially designed to deter these insects. Always make sure your room is well-ventilated if you use insecticides indoors.
> 'Cockroach traps' are available and can be placed in their favoured areas, such as near dustbins, under the sink or behind the refrigerator.

KEY FACTS

* Wasp, bee and mosquito stings can lead to violent allergic reactions.

* Don't forget cockroaches: their excrement can also cause adverse reactions in some people.

06

air your home

The air we breathe contains essential oxygen, but also dangerous pollutants, including carbon monoxide, irritants and allergens. To be certain of breathing clean air indoors, you must air your rooms regularly.

There is more to air than you might think

The air in your home contains various kinds of dust, allergenic substances left by house-dust mites and animals (see Tips 3 and 7), pollens (during spring and summer), combustion gases (carbon monoxide, sulphur dioxide) and fumes from varnish, paint, electrical appliances and cleaning products. Sometimes these substances are joined by mould that

● ● ● DID YOU KNOW? ──────────

> Ventilation systems can be installed reasonably easily.

> Centralized ventilation systems can be installed throughout your home or in certain key rooms. Air extractors continuously remove polluted air, which is then recycled.

> If you are highly allergic, you can install an independent ventilation unit in your bedroom.

> Heat-recovery ventilation systems are available that enable you to reuse the warm air from your kitchen and

has developed as a result of damp and moisture in bathrooms and kitchens (see Tip 8).

When all these substances combine, the result can be disastrous for a sensitive person. An allergic reaction causes inflammation (in the bronchial tubes, the skin, the nasal mucous membranes and so on), and these irritants simply exacerbate it.

Insulation equals pollution

The answer is simple: you need to ensure that your home is well aired. This means keeping the windows of an average-sized room wide open for five to ten minutes at least twice a day. Air all your rooms in this way, irrespective of the season, but avoid the times of day when flowers, trees and grasses are most actively releasing their pollen (early morning and late afternoon).

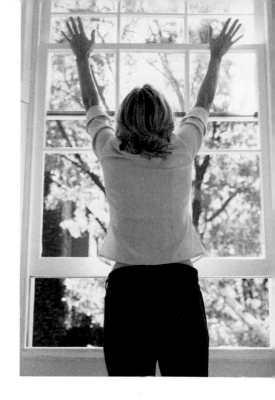

bathroom in your living rooms, after it has been filtered. Preferably choose a double-filter system that can eliminate both fumes and the tiniest particles.

KEY FACTS

* The air that we breathe in our homes contains allergens, harmful gases, mould spores, dust and pollen.

* Regularly air all your rooms and, if necessary, install a ventilation system.

07

say goodbye to house-dust mites

House-dust mites are microscopic arthropods, related to spiders. They live in our homes and are really bad news for most allergy sufferers. For example, between 60 and 90 per cent of all allergic asthma cases are caused by their faeces. But you can get rid of them.

Humidity, heat and skin

House-dust mites reproduce at an astonishing rate. It takes only six weeks for ten pairs of the creatures to create a colony of several thousand, provided they enjoy ideal conditions.

House-dust mites live off the flakes of dead skin that we shed continuously. This accumulates in bedding, soft furnishings and fitted carpets. There is little we can do about shedding our skin; however, mites are able to reproduce to their full potential only if they are also provided with heat and damp. A temperature of 22°C (72°F) and 75-80 per cent humidity constitute ideal conditions for these microscopic nasties.

Urgent measures

So your first step should be to reduce the humidity and heat by airing your bedroom well and turning down your central heating. You could also use a dehumidifier.

Furthermore, house-dust mites don't like ultraviolet rays, so regularly hang out your sheets, duvets and blankets to expose them to sunlight. Change your sheets frequently: twice a week if you're highly allergic. Don't forget to wash them at a high temperature: this will kill the mites. Finally, it's better to opt for blankets, pillows and duvets made of synthetic materials.

that have mainly natural active constituents, such as chrysanthemum flower extract. They are available in several forms: for the laundry, for carpets and for pillows (as an aerosol spray).

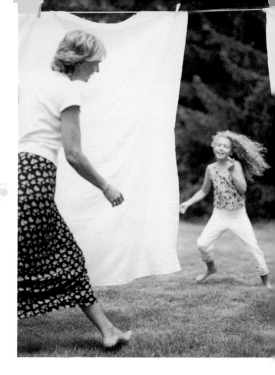

KEY FACTS

* House-dust mites like heat and humidity, so air your bedroom regularly and keep it cool at night.

* Change your sheets often and wash them in very hot water.

* Soft toys also provide a refuge for house-dust mites. You can kill them by sticking the teddy in the freezer for a day or two.

banish damp
from your home

Most domestic activities produce damp, a wonderful breeding ground for different types of mould, whose spores are very allergenic. To eliminate them, first locate the moulds and then stop future damp patches from forming.

● ● ● DID YOU KNOW?
> Dehumidifiers reduce dampness indoors by cooling the air so that the water particles in it condense.

> The water is collected in a container which can then be emptied out.
> Electrical dehumidifiers are more efficient than mechanical ones and require less maintenance.

Humidity and sustenance

Spores from mould are just like pollens: they spread in the air and cause allergic reactions. In our homes, they are, of course, mainly found in damp places (around the edges of the shower or bath, on kitchen furniture, around pipes, on porous walls, in cracks and so on).
To survive and grow, these moulds (such as Aspergillus and Penicilium) need a constant level of at least 70 per cent humidity and a regular supply of food. They get nourishment from cellulose materials, such as paints, wallpapers and textile wall-coverings. They're also fond of waste food and dust. So, to eradicate mould, you need to prevent your home from becoming damp and must keep all its nooks and crannies spotlessly clean.

Practical advice that really works

Firstly, check the places where moisture is liable to accumulate, such as around the edges of the shower and bath, and in sinks and washbasins. As soon as you see a dark mark, clean it with bleach. White vinegar also disinfects and cleans effectively. Next, check all the places where moisture might penetrate, or has already penetrated, from the outside (doors, windows, damp marks on the walls) and, if necessary, have them repaired or treated. Finally, make sure you clean very thoroughly all those places where damp and food debris might accumulate without being noticed, for instance, under electrical appliances, at the backs of kitchen cupboards and so on.

KEY FACTS

* Damp air indoors encourages the growth of mould that releases highly allergenic spores into the air.

* To stop moulds from forming, clean very damp areas with bleach or white vinegar.

* You could also install a dehumidifier in the rooms most susceptible to damp.

> Make sure you empty the water container regularly. Stagnant water encourages the growth of mould.

09

wage war on dust

Some people are allergic to dust or, more precisely, to various substances contained in these tiny particles, which get all over the house. You must be merciless against this microscopic enemy.

The downside of airing

Dust contains a wide range of substances, some of which (house-dust mite faeces, tiny pieces of cat's hair or bird's down, pollen from outdoors, smoke deposits) cause allergic reactions. No house is free from dust: it enters through doors, windows, gaps in the floorboards and partitions. And there's nothing you can do to stop it. What's more, it's a sad paradox that the more you air your

●●● DID YOU KNOW? ─────────

> If you are extremely allergic to dust, don't ever do your housework without taking some precautions.

> Put on a respiratory mask (a disposable surgical mask made of non-woven material; suitable designs are available on the Internet or from specialist suppliers) to reduce the amount of dust particles you inhale.

> Wear protective glasses if your eyes are sensitive.

> Wear gloves if contact with detergents causes you to develop skin allergies.

home to improve its air quality (see Tip 6), the more dust you allow inside. There's only one solution, and unfortunately it involves housework. You must dust your home frequently.

Lose that feather duster

Don't use a feather duster, because it disturbs the dust and simply gets it airborne again, allowing it to spread. Extra vigorous sweeping of a hard floor has the same effect. On hard surfaces (tiling, varnished wood, and so on) use a lightly damp floor cloth and rinse it regularly so it doesn't spread dust back on to the floor. For fitted carpets and rugs use an efficient vacuum cleaner (see Tip 11). Use a lightly damp cloth for dusting furniture. Some cleaning products even attract dust to the cloth. Check their ingredients, however, as some of them (especially the aerosols) contain irritants. Steam cleaners get rid of ingrained dust, but you should not need them if you dust your home regularly: at least twice a week. And don't reserve your spring cleaning for just once a year: give your home a thorough clean at least once a month. If you are highly allergic, get your partner to do the vacuuming and dusting.

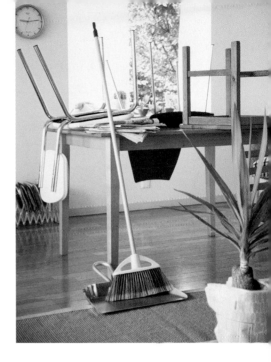

 KEY FACTS

* Dust contains several allergens, including house-dust mites, cat's hairs and mould spores.

* To eradicate dust, use a damp cloth or steam cleaners.

* Wear a respiratory mask when doing your housework and possibly protective gloves and glasses.

10

no more carpets and curtains

Fitted carpets and rugs, thick curtains and wall-hangings are all breeding-grounds for allergens. In bedrooms they provide a home around the bed for mites and they gather dust in living rooms. In damp rooms they attract moisture and mould. The best course of action is to get rid of them.

Wooden flooring, linoleum and tiles

Rugs and fitted carpets are real dust traps, so it's a good idea to replace them with hard materials, in which the dust can't accumulate. Uncovered boards are more suitable for rooms that are frequently occupied, such as bedrooms and living rooms. Varnished wooden flooring is much easier to maintain, as it can be washed and even cleaned with hygienic chlorine.

●●● DID YOU KNOW?

> The soles of our shoes bring in a host of unwelcome guests, such as pollen, mould and dust. Remove your shoes at the door and ask your visitors to do the same.

> Keep a collection of slippers lined up at the front door so that visitors may take off their shoes as soon as they arrive. Remember never to go outside in your slippers.

Avoid using lino or vinyl flooring in kitchens and bathrooms (mould can develop underneath it), as well as uncovered boards (they are almost impossible to make completely watertight). Floor tiles are a better option.

Blinds and double glazing

Wooden or plastic window blinds are preferable to curtains. They are easy to clean, because dust gathers on the slats and can be removed easily with a damp cloth (or a special brush). Blinds made of fabric, which create a warmer atmosphere, could also be fitted, provided the material is synthetic and has minimal folds and recesses.

Finally, double glazing gives several advantages: it reduces condensation and prevents mould from forming where the glass meets the window frame.

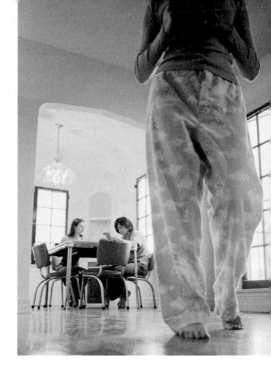

> If you can't do without fitted carpets, make sure that they've been treated against house-dust mites and mould, and vacuum them thoroughly on a regular basis.

 KEY FACTS

* Dust and allergens gather in fitted carpets, rugs, wall-coverings and curtains.

* For the floors, choose wooden flooring or tiling.

* Double glazing and blinds are best for windows.

11

choose a good vacuum cleaner

It's your number-one anti-dust weapon. However, some vacuum cleaners are much better than others. Allergy sufferers would do well to invest in a sophisticated model, capable of sucking up the tiniest particles, even those ensconced in the deepest armchairs.

In the morning

The more powerful a vacuum cleaner's motor, the more capacity it has to suck up large quantities of dust. The older types of machine are equipped with filters that can capture only the largest particles. House-dust mite faeces, for example, pass through them and back into the air again. Don't vacuum in the evening before going to bed to avoid inhaling particles suspended in the air

● ● ● DID YOU KNOW?

> Central vacuum systems are now increasingly available. The motor and dust container are kept in a storage room, such as a cellar or box-room, and the vacuum pipe is plugged into a socket in the room to be cleaned.

> These systems have several advantages: they are easy to use; the dust container is large and needs to be emptied only two or three times a year (preferably by someone who doesn't suffer from dust allergies);

while you sleep. If possible, do the job in the morning, with the windows open.

How to choose the ideal vacuum cleaner

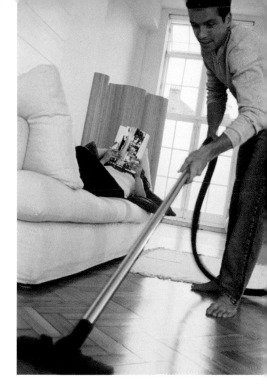

There are several points to consider when looking for a good vacuum cleaner. Firstly, power: the more powerful the machine, the more tiny particles of dust it will suck up . You can tell how powerful it is from its wattage. Today, there are plenty of vacuum cleaners of 1,000 watts or more. The next criterion is the quality of the filter: machines with a HEPA filter can capture the smallest particles, like house-dust mites' faeces and pollens. When buying, make sure that the system enables you to avoid contact with any dust when emptying the bag or changing the filter. Finally, check that the cleaner comes with the necessary accessories, such as brushes and nozzles for cleaning upholstery.

some systems are equipped with ventilation, which ejects the air that has been sucked in once all the dust has been removed.

KEY FACTS

* A good vacuum cleaner must be powerful enough to suck up tiny dust particles even from less accessible places.

* It must be equipped with a HEPA filter.

* Central vacuum systems are also available.

12 neat, tidy and simple

The more knick-knacks you have in your home, the more likely you are to suffer from allergies. That's because they all attract dust. So take your courage in both hands and get rid of all the things you don't need.

Dust thoroughly on top and underneath
The best way of stopping dust from accumulating is to clean and tidy your home regularly. Dust thoroughly and ensure every item is lifted to clean underneath it, and every piece of furniture should be moved to dust behind it. This is much easier to do if you have binned all your useless items. Get rid of all the little ornaments, souvenirs and other bits and pieces that clutter up shelves and the tops of cabinets.

Choose your furniture wisely
Put your books and CDs on shelves with glass panels: dust won't be able to gather on them and they'll be kept in pristine condition. Bookcases and cupboards are much easier to clean if they go right up to the ceiling; then they don't have any tops to clean. Be minimalist when furnishing your bedroom: the less clutter, the better you'll be able to sleep and the less likely you'll be to suffer any allergic reactions.

●●● DID YOU KNOW?

> Avoid all over-elaborate objects and furnishings: cabinets with decorative moulded edges and friezes, chandeliers, intricately decorated ornaments.

> Think twice before fitting any dust-gathering mouldings to walls, ceilings and skirting boards.

KEY FACTS

∗ Make your rooms easy to dust: don't clutter them up with ornaments, books and CDs and keep them tidy.

∗ Choose the minimalist approach to furnishing.

13 give up using detergents

Washing powders and other household cleaners can cause allergic reactions. If that happens to you, try some traditional methods instead.

Eczema and dermatitis Many strong chemicals and detergents leach grease from the skin causing a simple irritant eczema. To someone with a contact allergy, detergents can cause more severe eczema or dermatitis. These two conditions may also interact: a chemical irritant dermatitis making a contact reaction more likely; and people with eczema are generally more sensitive to irritants. The simplest solution is to simply give up using chemical detergents. If this is impossible, wear cotton-lined gloves and use barrier and emollient creams.

Tried and tested alternatives If you have a reaction to a household cleaner or detergent, first try other similar products. You might find one that doesn't irritate your skin. Organic cleaners should contain fewer irritants than their chemical-rich counterparts. Don't forget traditional methods: clean brass with a lemon; use eau de Cologne on coffee rings.

● ● ● DID YOU KNOW?

> Avoid perfumed products. They contain chemical compounds with strong irritant and allergenic effects.
> Choose less sophisticated products. They may lack the pleasant smell, but they should also lack unpleasant consequences.
> If you suffer from dish-pan hands, consider buying a dishwasher.

KEY FACTS

∗ Some people suffer from irritant and contact allergies when using cleaning products and detergents.

∗ Test out different brands, try organic products and, if all else fails, use traditional methods: vinegar, lemon juice, salt and so on.

14

take care when redecorating

Are you about to redecorate your home? If so, take care when choosing paint, wallpaper, varnishes and so on. If you follow a few simple guidelines, you'll have fewer and less serious allergic reactions.

On walls and woodwork

Paints and varnishes often contain a huge number of volatile organic compounds (VOCs). These are solvents that evaporate rapidly and emit irritant fumes for a long time after they have dried. Formaldehyde, for example, is widely used in chipboard panels, insulating foam, adhesives and varnishes. All of

● ● ●   D I D   Y O U   K N O W ?

> If you want to put up wallpaper, choose a very smooth, washable type, which is simple to clean.
> Wallpaper adhesives usually contain a fungicide to prevent the growth of mould under the paper, but, even so, be especially careful with moist, cold walls: the moisture could condense and become a breeding-ground for invisible mould.

these products can continue to emit toxic fumes for fifteen years after use. Glycol ethers, frequently found in paint, are equally harmful, as is pentachlorophenol, a fungicide that is often used in wood-treatment products.

Ecological paints and vegetable adhesives

Oil-based paint contains more VOCs than water-based. Ecological paints contain neither heavy metals (brass, lead, copper, zinc, etc.) nor glycol ethers.
Also available are anti-allergic paints and varnishes, which are totally free from VOCs. Look out for lime or mineral paints; paints with a base of proteins; or vegetable or synthetic resin.
To affix floor tiles or wall coverings, choose vegetable adhesives with a latex base that are free from solvents.

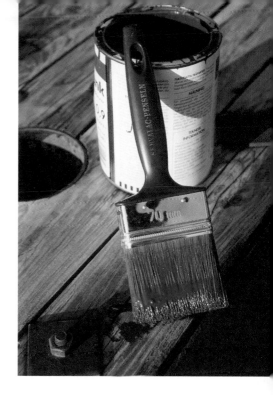

> Finally, if you opt for wood panelling, make sure you use good-quality adhesive, and don't put wooden slats on panels containing formaldehyde.

KEY FACTS

* If you want to redecorate your home, choose the products with care.

* Above all, avoid any products containing VOCs.

* Choose vegetable adhesives for fixing floor tiles and wall-coverings.

15 keep an eye on your diet

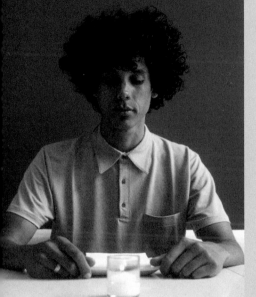

Increasing numbers of people are suffering from food allergies. Some foodstuffs can cause severe reactions, particularly in young children. This problem needs to be given special consideration because these allergies can affect the whole body and provoke many reactions.

How do allergens enter the body?

Allergens penetrate the body in a variety of ways: via the respiratory tract, the eyes, the skin or the throat. The allergic reaction occurs either in the place of contact, as happens with contact eczema and conjunctivitis caused by pollen, or in the bloodstream.

Food allergies are the most insidious, because they can cause reactions in many different parts of the body.

It starts in childhood

Young children are the most susceptible to food allergies. Even some breast-fed babies can develop an allergy if the milk contains allergenic proteins from the mother's diet. In most cases, if a close eye is kept on what the child eats during the first few years, the allergy will decrease in severity and disappear altogether before the age of ten.

sensitive stomach that reacts much more than normal to products that are not fresh or that contain chemical substances.

It has been established that if both parents are allergy sufferers, a child has a 50 per cent chance of being one, too. There is a 33 per cent possibility if only one parent is allergic, and hardly more than 10 per cent if neither is. If both parents have allergies, doctors advise that the child should be breast-fed for its first three months. Food most likely to cause allergies, such as eggs and milk from animals, must not be given before the child is one year old.

Consult your doctor to discuss what foods you can safely give your child while ensuring they have a healthy diet.

KEY FACTS

* Food allergies cause whole-body reactions, sometimes very severe ones.

* Children, and sometimes even babies, are more affected than adults.

* A food allergy should not be confused with food intolerance, although the two reactions can occur at the same time.

16

eat organic food

People who suffer from food allergies are particularly sensitive to some chemical ingredients, which can sometimes cause severe reactions. The best way of avoiding food additives and colouring agents is to eat organic food.

Allergic reaction enhancers

Manufactured foods all contain chemical substances: preservatives, sweeteners, thickening agents, flavour enhancers, colourings, antioxidants, etc. They cause allergic reactions in some people, while others, who are already especially sensitive to the food, experience more severe symptoms because of the additives. Eating organic food is a good way to deal with this problem. To avoid additives,

● ● ● D I D   Y O U   K N O W ?

> Organic medicinal herbs are also available. If you have to take a course of herbal medicine, which some allergies require, or if you just like a cup of herbal tea in the evening, why not try them?

> Just like other organic foodstuffs, they are never subjected to chemical treatments or irradiation.
> They must be dried and stored in premises built with materials that do not emit harmful fumes. Even the

avoid prepared foods such as TV dinners or pies, buy fresh fruit, vegetables and meat, and cook for yourself.

Organic is best, but not infallible

Nowadays, there are all kinds of organic foods on offer: fresh (meat, vegetables, eggs, milk and dairy products), frozen (particularly meat and vegetables), even processed foods (pasta, biscuits, etc.). They are often identified by a symbol, which may vary from country to country, but which is always only awarded after rigorous checks by official organizations. The symbol indicates that the product meets all the specifications of organic farming and/or stockbreeding.

A word of warning: switching to organic does not mean that you can now safely eat food that you have reacted to in the past. If, for example, you are allergic to peanuts, you will still react to those even with an organic logo on the packet.

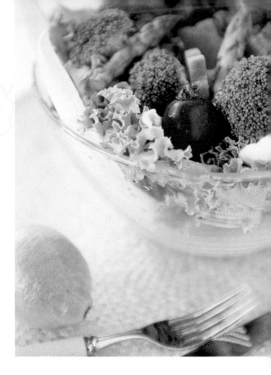

beams that are used in the construction of store-rooms must not be treated with chemical fungicides.

> Again, a specific logo will act as a guarantee that no chemical residue is liable to be lurking in the bottom of your cup.

KEY FACTS

* Food additives can cause or exacerbate allergic reactions.

* To avoid them, the best idea is to eat organic food.

* Organic foods are clearly labelled, and must meet very strict criteria before they can display that label.

17

The most common food allergies are those caused by peanuts, cow's milk, wheat, eggs, fish, shellfish and strawberries. But children and adults don't tend to react to the same foods.

peanuts, milk, strawberries, shellfish...

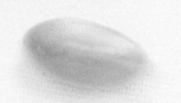

To every age its allergies

Much research has taken place all over the world to try to identify the foods that most commonly cause allergies. Check out the Internet for more information or look in the library for specific books on the subject.

Among adults: top of the list were fruits belonging to the Rosaceae family (plums, strawberries), followed by those

●●● DID YOU KNOW?

> Gluten intolerance is not, strictly speaking, an allergy, although the immune system is involved.

> It is an autoimmune illness that affects the digestive system, sometimes seriously: it can cause nausea, vomiting, diarrhoea, bloating and stomach pains.

> Gluten is a protein found in cereals, and therefore in pasta, bread and cakes, but also, among other things, in fish coated with breadcrumbs, numerous mass-produced cooked products, many sauces, some milk desserts and beer.

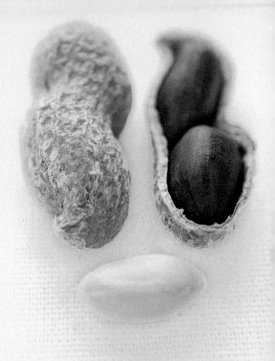

belonging to the latex group (avocados, bananas, kiwi fruits), umbelliferous plants (parsley, carrots, sunflower), dried fruit, egg white, sesame, peanuts and shellfish.

Among children: first came allergies caused by egg white, followed by peanuts, cow's milk, fish, walnuts and shellfish.
If your child develops a food allergy, pay close attention to what they eat. Begin by removing from their diet all foods well known for being allergenic (those listed above). Then reintroduce them one by one at intervals of a few days. Remember, though, children have different dietary needs from adults, and you may need advice from a dietician to make sure that an exclusion diet is still nutritionally complete.

> The only effective way of dealing with the problem is to avoid all foods containing gluten. 'Gluten-free' products, including jars of baby food, are on sale in health-food shops and increasingly in supermarkets.

KEY FACTS

* Children and adults are not sensitive to the same foods.

* Among children, the foods that cause most allergic reactions are egg whites, peanuts and cow's milk.

* In adults, the main culprits are strawberries, kiwi fruits, bananas and avocados, as well as peanuts, eggs and fish.

18

go to the dentist's

Some research suggests that allergies could be the result of long-term poisoning by mercury in traditional dental fillings. This is a controversial theory, and, naturally, the dental community denies it vehemently, but, if you are concerned, there are steps you can take.

Mercury

Of course, not all allergies can be blamed on fillings. Yet some difficult-to-treat allergic reactions could be the result of slow mercury poisoning. Most of the European scientific and medical communities are reluctant to accept this, but in some countries, such as Japan and Sweden, the use of such fillings has been discontinued.

Mercury salts are extremely toxic when either inhaled or swallowed, but in dental fillings the mercury is combined with other metals: fillings usually weigh about 2g, roughly half of which is mercury. In the past, these compounds were thought to be perfectly stable and leakages were thought impossible, even after years of use. However, recent studies have shown that leaks of mercury vapours and ions might occur. Much of the evidence still

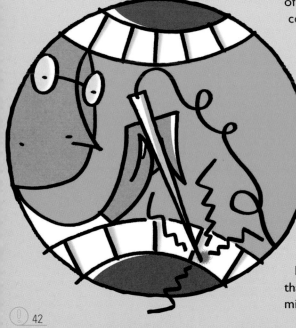

remains contradictory and inconclusive, and some researchers have suggested that mercury in the body is more likely to come from diet than dental fillings.

Headaches, tiredness and allergies

Those campaigning against mercury fillings claim that some people are more sensitive than others to these leaks, due to the chemical composition of their saliva and the interaction with other substances in the mouth. People who are highly susceptible are said to experience headaches, chronic fatigue and allergy attacks. If you suffer allergic reactions but don't know their cause, it might be worthwhile consulting a sympathetic dentist. You could have your fillings replaced with porcelain or gold inlays, glass ionomer cement or resin fillings, or even, in certain cases, dental implants.

Remember, though, this should not be entered into lightly. First, it is expensive. Second, if you remove your fillings, you may reawaken dormant infections. Third, most people find going to the dentist stressful. Finally, your dentist will probably have to enlarge the existing cavity to provide a good base for the new filling, so you lose more of your own tooth.

If you decide to go ahead and have your old fillings removed, this must be done in carefully controlled conditions, as a large amount of mercury vapour is released during the procedure.

● ● ● DID YOU KNOW?

> On contact with the saliva, mercury vapours are thought to escape from dental fillings and are inhaled, causing, over a long period of time, allergic reactions that are difficult to cure.

> Food supplements such as selenium and vitamin C protect the body against the harmful effects of mercury.

> Mercury is 25 times more toxic than arsenic.

KEY FACTS

* Mercury is very toxic, but much less so when bound with other metals in amalgam.

* Dental fillings may release poisonous mercury vapours and ions.

* If you have allergies that you can't seem to cure, consult a dentist sympathetic to the problem, who might advise replacement of your amalgam fillings.

19

consult your doctor

You must see your doctor if you have an allergy. It should not be considered unimportant, even when the symptoms are not severe. Before deciding what should be done about it, you need to know the reason for your allergy and the range of treatments available.

First and foremost, get a diagnosis

Allergies are not harmless, and the many forms they take can make it difficult to work out the exact cause of the problem. Only a doctor is really in a position to understand the symptoms, make a firm diagnosis and, possibly, carry out tests to identify the guilty allergen or allergens.

Then it's up to you to handle the illness on a daily basis. However serious your allergy, a healthy lifestyle will always help matters and, in some cases, be enough to put things right. In others, it will improve the effectiveness of any drugs that have been prescribed.

The most frequently used treatments

Antihistamines are frequently prescribed for allergic rhinitis (hay fever) and conjunctivitis. They reduce the production of histamine, which is responsible for allergic symptoms. Antihistamines used to be notorious for causing drowsiness, but this has now largely been eradicated. Nasal sprays and anti-inflammatory eye drops are also widely available to alleviate the symptoms of hay fever.

Treatment of asthma has been revolutionized by the use of bronchodilators, which rapidly relax the muscles in the bronchial passages and relieve the sensation of suffocation.

Corticosteroids are widely used as creams for eczema, as nose drops in cases of allergic rhinitis and as inhaled treatments to suppress inflammation of the airways in asthma. By giving corticosteroids topically in this way, there is less absorption into the body as a whole, so reducing side-effects and improving both their efficiency and the patient's ability to tolerate them.

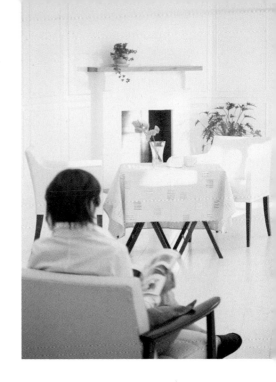

KEY FACTS

* Allergies should not be taken lightly, even when the symptoms are not severe.

* Your doctor will be able to carry out tests to discover what is causing the allergy.

* Drug treatment should also be accompanied by a healthy lifestyle.

20 dealing with emergencies

The possibility that an allergy sufferer might have a very severe and sudden reaction can never be ruled out entirely. So be prepared; you never know.

Severe reactions The major dangers are anaphylactic shock, which can seriously affect the whole body, and angioedema (such as hives, weals or nettle rash) with swelling, often around the eyes, lips and hands. Swelling in the mouth or larynx can cause suffocation. Both angioedema and anaphylaxis can develop very rapidly, usually after the patient has been stung by an insect or has consumed something, like peanuts or a drug, that causes a powerful allergic reaction.

Tingling lips and a swollen tongue If your lips tingle, your tongue feels swollen and rashes suddenly appear, call for medical help immediately. If you are with someone suffering from these symptoms and they lose consciousness, lay them on their side and wait for help to arrive. If the problem seems to be throat oedema, keep the patient in a seated position so that it's easier for them to breathe.

KEY FACTS

* Anaphylactic shock and angioedema are very serious allergic reactions that require the help of emergency medical services.

* The main initial signs are tingling lips, swollen tongue, breathlessness and nausea.

case study

Life's good, despite my allergy

« It happened one spring day, when I was enjoying a picnic with my parents in the countryside. I was nearly fifteen. I started to sneeze and couldn't stop, my nose kept running and my eyes kept watering. An hour later I was having difficulty breathing and my eyes were so swollen that I couldn't open them. I discovered I was allergic to grass pollen! I suffered the same symptoms in the middle of each spring for some years. Then I began to react to other things: I couldn't sleep on feather pillows any more, or smell flowers, or stroke cats. I had to adapt. I learnt to avoid certain spots at certain times of the year, to go on holiday to places where I wouldn't be affected by my allergies and always to take my synthetic pillow with me when I was away from home. Over the years the symptoms have become less acute. Nowadays I can live with my allergy. I don't often get attacks, but when I do feel them coming on, I quickly realize what's caused the reaction and move away from it. When all is said and done, that's the best thing to do. »

21 >>>

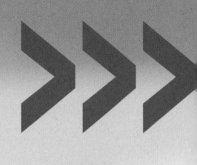

>> **Many allergic reactions occur in the respiratory tract.** Among the most common are hay fever and asthma, which tend to run in families. Hay fever, an allergic reaction to pollen, is characterized by rhinitis and conjunctivitis. The allergic reactions in asthma occur in the airways, with pollen just one of many potential triggers.

>>>> In addition to the drugs you take to regulate your immune system, **there are natural methods of treating allergy symptoms**, such as homeopathy, herbs, exercise and relaxation.

>>>>>> To stop your allergy attacks, or at least to make your drugs work more effectively, **you can practise exercises** that can be performed at the times of day that suit you best.

40
TIPS

21

treat your symptoms

If you suffer from asthma, hay fever or conjunctivitis, you must certainly try to discover which allergen is to blame and attempt to control your immune system's excessive response to it. But you still need to relieve your symptoms. Here we look at the effects of these three allergies.

Is your nose running?

An allergen disturbs the immune system, which then produces localized symptoms. The nature of the allergen needs to be addressed, as do the symptoms. Hay fever (or allergic rhinitis) often starts very suddenly. First, you get a runny nose that is usually accompanied by bursts of violent sneezing. Your eyes and nose feel itchy, and if this extends to your throat, you start to suffer from a dry cough. The symptoms can stop as suddenly as they began, as soon as the allergen responsible disappears.

If it is persistent, hay fever can also cause inflammation and infections in the ears and sinuses, especially if you also suffer from a cold or other viral infection.

Do you find it hard to breathe?

The other allergic symptom affecting the respiratory tract is asthma. This narrowing of the bronchial airways is affecting increasing numbers of people in the Western world each year.

You start to find it difficult to breathe, as if your bronchial tubes have been blocked, and feel as if your chest is being gripped by a vice. Your chest muscles contract to expel the air in your lungs but struggle to do so because of the narrowed bronchial airways. You gasp for breath. The membranes lining the bronchial walls secrete tenacious mucus, which congests the airways even further. You might experience tightness in the chest and wheeze, or you might suffer from a troublesome dry cough which turns into paroxysms of coughing triggered by moving, talking or even just inhaling, and which keeps you awake at night. Apart from allergies, viral infections like the common cold might trigger an episode of asthma in people who are susceptible.

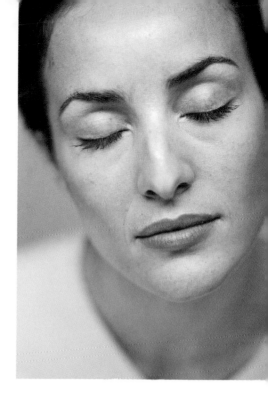

KEY FACTS

* Treating an allergy also involves relieving its symptoms.

* Hay fever causes watery eyes, a runny nose and sneezing.

* Asthma causes breathing difficulties due to narrowing of the bronchial tubes.

22

take a kinesiology test

This therapy, based upon the concept of the body's energy flow, can trace the allergen responsible for your problems and, what's more, teach your body to accept it. Not everybody is convinced by the technique, but it has its followers and can boast some undeniable successes.

Dr Goodheart's discovery

In 1964, when the American chiropractor Dr Goodheart was studying Chinese medicine, he noticed a close affinity between certain muscles and acupuncture meridians and thus with the organs associated with them. This gave him the idea of testing or 'questioning' the strength of these muscles to obtain responses from the energy flow.

● ● ● DID YOU KNOW?

> Kinesiology is also concerned with healing. In this therapy, just as in traditional Chinese medicine, it is believed that all illnesses originate from a disturbance in the energy flow: the visible symptoms are only an outward sign of this.

> The kinesiologist 'reprogrammes' the body, removing all trace of the allergic sensitivity by correcting the circulation of energy. This is done simply by gentle manipulation of acupuncture points.

His kinesiology tests are now well known. They are based on the simple fact that when you hold your arm out straight, your muscles tense. This tension can be weakened by many factors, such as stress or a joint problem. It is also weakened in response to messages from the energy flow. According to exponents of kinesiology, the body 'recognizes' messages from the energy flow about substances likely to cause it illnesses.

Allergens in little bottles

To give an example: you stand with your arm stretched out and the kinesiologist puts a little bottle containing a very toxic substance in your hand. Your energy flow 'recognizes' the toxicity of the substance and your muscles weaken. If the therapist puts his hand on your arm, your arm will be able to put up very little resistance and will give way.

The same procedure is followed when testing for allergies, except that the little bottles are filled with allergens, such as animal hairs, pollen and dust. When you are holding the bottle containing the allergen that you react to, your arm will lose its strength and give way. This is a very simple way of tracing the allergens you should avoid.

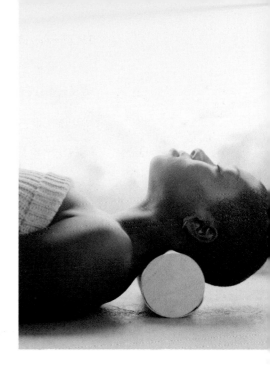

KEY FACTS

* Kinesiology is based on the same principle as traditional Chinese medicine: a disruption in the energy flow is the cause of allergies.

* A very simple muscle test identifies the allergens and gentle manipulative movements 'reprogramme' the circulation of energy.

23

try homeopathy

Homeopathy is a highly effective method of treating allergies, especially respiratory problems. To a homeopathic doctor, each patient is unique and requires individual treatment. Homeopaths have galleries of patient-types to help them understand the patient's personality and background.

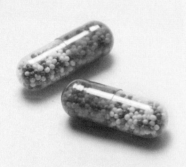

Each patient is different

Homeopathy does not treat an illness but a sick individual. For example, more than a dozen homeopathic remedies are currently available to treat the common cold, and the doctor will not only choose the one that best fits your symptoms, but also your personality and behaviour. The sum of all these characteristics is called your 'terrain'. This idea is particu-

● ● ● DID YOU KNOW?

> These portraits were developed at the same time as homeopathy itself.
> Its founder, Samuel Hahnemann, noticed that an extremely diluted substance cured symptoms that it would promote if adminis-

tered in a concentrated form. For example, diluted coffee cured the insomnia caused by too much coffee.
> Hahnemann tested all the medicines available at the time and noted

larly relevant when treating allergies, because each person's allergic reactions differ. To achieve a better understanding of the sick person's 'terrain', a homeopathic practitioner will often refer to 'portraits' or homeopathic types, which are associated with the main remedies.

Aconite, Pulsatilla, Lycopodium

• Aconite type patients, for example, are often frightened of crowds. The slightest stress is too much for them. They have a great fear of death. If they are allergic, their allergies usually cause respiratory symptoms and their asthma attacks are particularly painful.
• Pulsatilla types are very emotional and cry over the slightest thing. They are very susceptible to infections and tend to suffer from congestion in the respiratory tract. They are likely to suffer from chronic hay fever that leads to inflammation and infection.

• Lycopodium types have a characteristically sluggish digestion. They find it hard to wake up in the mornings and you should never try to make conversation with them over breakfast! They are rather pessimistic and tend to keep themselves to themselves. When it comes to allergies, they are likely to suffer stomach or skin reactions.

When the doctor finds the type you most closely resemble, he will prescribe the corresponding remedy to cure the flaws of your basic 'terrain'.

their effects to find out which ones had a therapeutic value when highly diluted.
> The portraits arose from the thorough observations of his patients, and homeopathic doctors still use them today.

KEY FACTS

∗ To a homeopathic doctor, each patient is unique.

∗ The homeopathic patient types are very useful to the doctor, especially when treating allergies, because everyone reacts to allergies in their own distinctive way.

24

the right treatments for asthma

A good homeopathic cure usually combines a basic treatment with an individualized crisis treatment appropriate to your symptoms. The remedies chosen to treat asthma depend on many factors, which only a doctor is in a position to appreciate fully.

Histamine in homeopathic doses

Poumon histamine is a dilution of histamine, designed to reduce the body's production of this substance. It is one of the fundamental homeopathic medicines for treating respiratory allergies.

The other remedies given depend upon your symptoms. If your asthma is 'dry' (accompanied by a dry cough), the remedy prescribed is Aconitum Napellus (if you suffer from anxiety), Spongia (if your nose and throat are very sensitive), Ipeca (if you are pale, have rings under your eyes and experience nausea) or Moschus (if at the same time you suffer attacks of tachycardia).

'Wet' asthma, when the attacks cause the production of mucus, usually calls for Coccus Cacti.

Making a physical effort

Some people have asthma attacks immediately after physical exercise (see Tip 32). The medicines that are suitable for this form of asthma are Ignatia and Cuprum Metallicum.

Children who suffer from asthma don't all receive the same treatment. Those who are quick-tempered and aggressive are often prescribed Chamomilla, while extremely sensitive children are given Causticum.

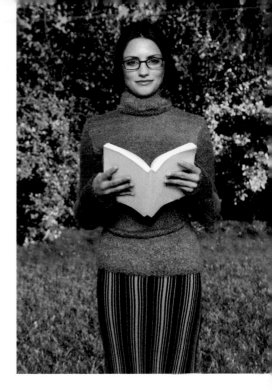

requires proper medical care. Make sure you consult a well-trained homeopathic doctor.

> Remember that homeopathy works gradually. While it might reduce the frequency of attacks over the long term, acute episodes of asthma require prompt treatment with conventional remedies, giving instant, possibly life-saving, results.

KEY FACTS

* A homeopathic cure combines a basic treatment with a crisis treatment.

* The latter is chosen according to your symptoms.

* Some medicines are suitable in particular for children who suffer from asthma.

25 stop sneezing

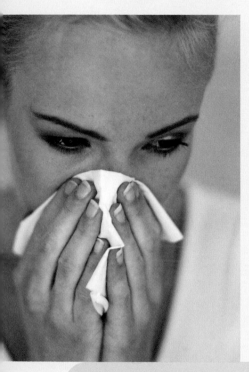

With its symptoms of streaming nose, sneezing fits and watery eyes, hay fever isn't a dangerous illness but it's a very uncomfortable one. Homeopathy can provide you with the individualized remedies to make you feel much better.

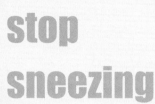

DID YOU KNOW?

> Respiratory allergies can lead to partial or total loss of sense of smell. This is called anosmia.

> If you have suffered from this for a long time, try Pulsatilla.
> If you are also suffering from a deviation of the nasal septum (abnormal position of the partition between the two nostrils), it is likely that a course of Sanguinaria will relieve the problem.

Does it tickle or itch?

With tissue permanently in hand, nose red, eyes weeping and ears blocked, hay fever sufferers often look a pitiful sight. And this very disruptive condition can sometimes last for weeks on end. To put a stop to these yearly attacks, most often due to pollen, doses of Pollen 30 HC, a dilution of several different pollens, are usually prescribed. After that, the choice of remedy depends on the exact nature of your reactions.

If your nose runs and your voice is hoarse but your eyes are fine, you will probably benefit from Allium Cepa, the homeopathic dilution of onion. If your palate and ears itch while your nose is running, you probably need to try Arundo Donax.

Bless you!

Other factors, such as sneezing, can then enter the equation. If you sneeze frequently and this gives rise to bouts of dry coughing, you will probably be prescribed Nathtalinum. If you are constantly sneezing and tire easily, feeling almost as if you have the flu, you will be helped by Pulsatilla, Hydrastis or Kalium Phosphoricum (should you feel better in a cool place) or Sabadilla, Nux Vomica or Kalium Muriaticum (should you feel better in a warm room).

> If your nose is blocked with a thick and sticky discharge as well, then choose Kalium Bichromicum.

KEY FACTS

* Hay fever is often very unpleasant for the sufferer.

* It can be treated with homeopathic remedies chosen according to the nature and amount of nasal discharge.

* Sneezing and loss of sense of smell can be relieved by other remedies.

26

disinfect the air around you

The air we breathe indoors is polluted by enormous numbers of irritants and contains thousands of bacteria and viruses. To be sure of avoiding all risk of infection, however slight, cleanse the air with essential oils.

Keeping the air pure

It is vital that people susceptible to respiratory allergies should breathe pure, healthy air. Otherwise, they risk infection, which will only exacerbate their respiratory problems. There is a simple, pleasant and effective way of doing this: spread essential oils throughout your home. These oils are highly concentrated extracts of aromatic herbs and have medicinal, often disinfectant and antibiotic, properties: they destroy bacteria when they come into direct contact with them.

Buy yourself a special diffuser. These are small, unobtrusive electrical devices into which you pour a few drops of a mixture of essential oils. The oils are then dispersed into the air in the form of microscopic droplets. Diffusers that don't heat the oils are best, because heating can deprive them of some of their valuable properties.

Choosing the right oils

Firstly, make up a mixture according to your personal preference: some oils smell very pleasant (lavender, neroli, sandalwood), while others (thyme, basil, bergamot) have strong, bracing scents. Test out the mixtures until you find a fragrance you really like.

Later, you might vary the oils according to the time of day: some oils (lemon, mint, vervein) have an invigorating effect and are more suited to mornings, while others (rosewood, camomile, jasmine) have sedative qualities that prepare you for a night's sleep.

Finally, there are some oils (eucalyptus, pine, oregano) that have a direct effect on the respiratory system by easing pulmonary inflammation and clearing the upper air passages.

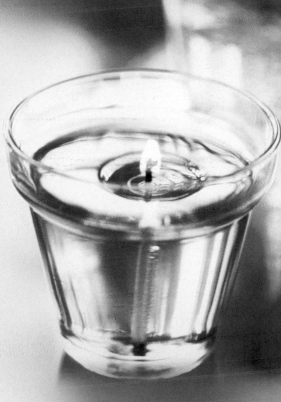

 KEY FACTS

* Dispersing essential oils is a simple, pleasant and effective way of disinfecting the air in your home.

* Choose the oils according to your preferences, the time of day and your particular health problems.

27

treat yourself with plants

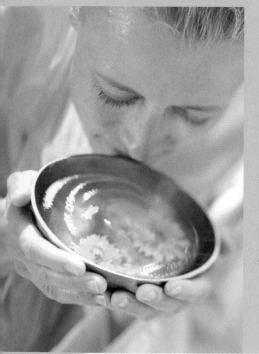

Medicinal plants can often gently and naturally relieve the symptoms of respiratory allergies. Marsh mallow, pine and violet, among others, soothe inflamed bronchial tubes and mucous membranes. Use them after attacks to speed up your recovery.

> They are both capable of soothing irritation and inflammation, and are often taken together.

●●● DID YOU KNOW?

> Two small, unassuming flowers, the violet and the speedwell, shouldn't be overlooked.

Marsh mallow, a soothing plant

This plant is a member of the Malvaceae family and grows particularly well in damp areas close to the sea. It contains a large amount of soothing mucilage, so it rapidly eases inflammation of the mucous membranes and lungs. Use its flowers and especially its roots, finely chopped, to make infusions. These are very effective in the relief of hay fever and help stubborn coughs.

To prepare your infusion (or herbal tea), use 30g (1oz) of roots and flowers for every litre (2 pints) of boiling water. Infuse for ten minutes before filtering. You can drink three large cupfuls, sweetened with honey, each day.

Pine for guaranteed relief

Pine-cone buds contain an essential oil that soothes irritation and inflammation, making it ideal for the relief of problems in the bronchial tubes and upper air passages caused by allergies: for example, bronchial congestion, resulting from moderate or minor asthma attacks, and hay fever. Pine also helps to prevent secondary infections from establishing themselves in tissues inflamed by allergic reactions.

To prepare a pine herbal tea, put 2 table-spoonfuls of buds into 500ml (1 pint) of cold water. Boil for five minutes with the lid on. Don't forget to collect the drops of water that have condensed on the lid, as they are the richest in the effective substances. Leave to cool and drink up to two lukewarm cups per day, sweetened with honey.

> Put 15g (¹/₂oz) of each flower into 1 litre (2 pints) of boiling water. Infuse for ten minutes, filter and sweeten with honey. Drink up to three cups each day.

KEY FACTS

* Some plants are excellent for soothing areas of the respiratory tract, such as the bronchial tubes and mucous membranes, inflamed by allergies.

* Marsh mallow and pine are two of the best.

* Violets and speedwell are also very effective.

28 a treat for sore eyes

If your eyes are irritated by pollen, dust or cat's hair, cornflower or red vine preparations can help you.

If your eyes won't stop watering The cornflower has been used for centuries to relieve eye irritations. This small, delicate blue flower has soothing qualities that are well known. To make an effective eye lotion, place 20g (³/₄ oz) of plantain leaves and 20g of cornflower flowers in 1 litre (2 pints) of cold water. Heat the mixture until it just starts to boil, then remove it from the hob and let it cool down completely. Filter the cooled liquid carefully, then use for compresses or as an eye lotion.

If your eyes are red Red vine has an excellent effect on blood circulation. It also relieves eye irritation by improving the blood flow in the intricate network of tiny blood vessels. To prepare a lotion, use 3 tablespoonfuls of red vine leaves for every 500ml (1 pint) of cold water. Heat until the water and leaves come to the boil, then remove from the hob, let it cool and filter. Use for compresses and eye lotions.

● ● ● DID YOU KNOW?

> **Bilberry is also good for the eyes, being astringent (stops bleeding), soothing and antiseptic.**
> **Put 2 tablespoonfuls of leaves and berries in 500ml (1 pint) of boiling water, infuse for 10 minutes, filter and use as an eye lotion.**

KEY FACTS

* The cornflower is renowned for its soothing qualities.

* Red vine relieves eye irritation by improving the blood flow in the eye's network of blood vessels.

29 discover acupuncture

Traditional Chinese medicine has its own remedies for allergies. The acupuncturist's needles can often work wonders.

It's all due to the liver According to Chinese medicine, most respiratory allergies are due to an energy imbalance in the liver. While in Western medicine the liver is simply an important component in the body's digestive system and powerful filter of waste matter, in traditional Chinese medicine it is the organ mainly responsible for controlling the circulation and distribution of energy in the body's various meridians (energy channels). It also controls our body's defences against the external world.

On the face or between the shoulder blades Allergies are therefore due to an excess of energy in the liver meridian. To cure this, the acupuncturist must disperse the unwanted accumulation by inserting needles along the course of the liver meridian. Specific points – on the face either side of the nose or between the shoulder blades – can be targeted to put a rapid end to the symptoms.

● ● ● DID YOU KNOW?

> There are some strange coincidences. In Chinese symbolism, the liver is associated with wood and springtime.

> Of course, a number of respiratory allergies are caused by tree pollens and occur in that particular season.

KEY FACTS

* In Chinese medicine it is thought that allergies are the result of an excess of energy in the liver meridian.

* To cure them, the acupuncturist places needles at points along the liver meridian, on the face or between the shoulder blades.

30

Self-massage is another method you can use to alleviate uncomfortable symptoms. Jin shin do is acupuncture without the needles. You can practise it on yourself, provided you locate the right points to massage.

give yourself a facial massage

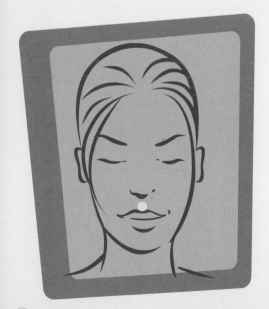

Clearing blocked air passages

Certain points on the body can be massaged to clear the air passages when they become blocked by a bronchial muscle spasm, which can sometimes happen during an asthma attack. Stimulating these points rapidly opens up the airways.

One of the points is on the back in the middle of a line running between the upper part of the two shoulder blades. You can massage the whole of this area, concentrating on any painful points. Another point, very easy to locate, lies just below the nose, in the middle of the philtrum (the furrow between the bottom of the nose and the upper lip).

Relieving hay fever

To ease the effects of hay fever, you can massage the points mentioned above, as well as several others: the hollow under the chin; the hollow where the two collarbones meet; and, especially, the wings of the nose. Spend a long time on this last point, moving up on both sides from the base of the nose to the eyes.

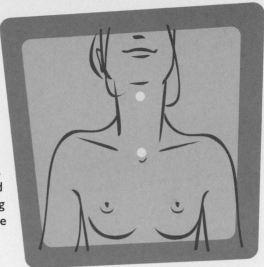

31
stop
smoking

Smoking is highly dangerous for everyone, especially for people who suffer from respiratory allergies. If you are a smoker, it's never too early to quit. It's never easy, but you will soon feel better for it.

A source of many extra toxins

Tobacco smoke contains a host of toxins and irritants capable of damaging anyone's respiratory system. So think what its tar, nicotine, carbon monoxide, ammonia and benzopyrene, among other substances, can do to someone whose nose, throat and lungs have already been weakened by respiratory allergies. What's more, nicotine accelerates the functions of the sympathetic nervous system, causing the

● ● ● DID YOU KNOW?

> If you've been a heavy smoker for a long time, it will take three months for your lungs to be restored to a healthy condition.

> However, eight hours after giving up, the level of carbon monoxide and nicotine in your bloodstream will already have declined by 50 per cent. After two days, your blood will be completely clear of them. After three days of total abstinence, the tissues in your lungs will be receiving more oxygen and starting the recovery process.

arteries to narrow, blood pressure to rise and the heart to beat faster, all factors that exacerbate asthma attacks.

Smoking does constant harm to the body and leads in the long term to the gravest of consequences: it is still one of leading causes of death in the Western world.

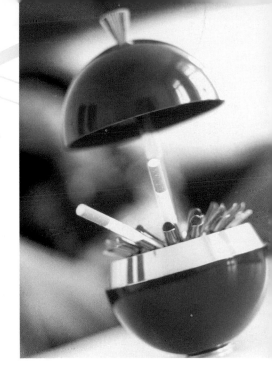

Herbal medicine, homeopathy, acupuncture

If you are a smoker, chances are you will already have tried to quit (maybe many times). However, if you are determined to stop poisoning yourself, help is at hand.

• Herbal medicine: some plants (valerian, passionflower) calm the nerves, others (eucalyptus, myrtle) help to clear the remains of tobacco from the bronchial passages, and others still (artichoke, meadowsweet) help the liver and kidneys to excrete toxins that have accumulated throughout the body.

• Homeopathy: appropriate treatment shortens the withdrawal period and reduces the craving.

• Acupuncture is very effective. You can lose the desire to smoke in one session. After that, it's a matter of will-power.

If these methods fail, then your doctor or pharmacist may be able to advise you about nicotine replacement therapy.

KEY FACTS

∗ Tobacco smoke is full of toxins and irritants.

∗ These substances irritate the bronchial passages, nose and throat of people who suffer from respiratory allergies.

∗ Complementary medicine can help you stop smoking.

32

get some exercise

For a long time it was thought that physical exercise was counter-productive for asthma sufferers. Now we know this is not true. Exercise can even be part of the treatment. What's more, some great sportspeople have had asthma. So why not follow their example?

Mountain climber, basketball player, diver

Catherine Destivelle used to suffer from asthma, but that hasn't stopped her from becoming one of the world's top climbers. Among other exploits, she undertook a solo ascent of the north face of the Drus, Mont Blanc, in ten days. Dennis Rodman, one of the stars of the all-conquering Chicago Bulls basketball

> It is acknowledged that asthma attacks can be triggered by strenuous exercise; typically the attack begins as the exercise ends.
> The inhalation of cold, dry air has also been shown to precipitate attacks, which may be due to the drying and cooling of the lining of the bronchi (airways).

> To avoid this risk, don't overdo your exercise, increase your efforts very gradually and, above all, warm up thoroughly before starting.
> In addition, if you're already feeling wheezy, exercise will exacerbate your breathlessness.

team in the 1990s, and Olympic diving champion Greg Louganis are both asthma sufferers, too.

Their examples prove that, far from being out of the question if you suffer from respiratory allergies, exercise is beneficial: it improves lung capacity, strengthens the cardiovascular system and helps to eliminate the stress that aggravates asthma attacks.

Beware of allergens indoors and out

On the other hand, allergy sufferers must be careful about where they exercise and which sports they pursue. Avoid sports that involve animals, such as horseriding. If your sport takes place outside, keep well away from all sources of allergens (trees with pollen, animals, dust, smoke and so on). If it is an indoor sport, make sure the room is well ventilated and free from damp and mould. If you choose a sport that takes place on a mat, such as gymnastics or judo, check that this is dusted regularly and thoroughly.

Swimming is a first-class exercise for asthmatics, but avoid swimming pools that put large quantities of chlorine in the water.

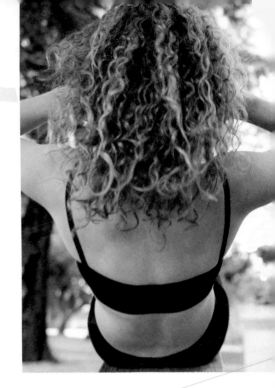

KEY FACTS

* Allergy sufferers, even those who have asthma, should take exercise.

* Many famous sportspeople are asthmatics.

* Exercise improves lung capacity, strengthens the cardiovascular system and reduces stress.

33 avoid stress

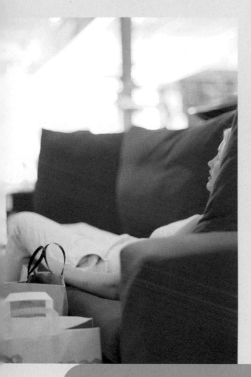

Stress affects everyone in the Western world, especially allergy sufferers. It has a direct effect on the immune system and increases its reactions, which is something all allergy sufferers need to avoid.

● ● ● DID YOU KNOW?

> Asthma can be caused by genetic factors, as with other allergies. If both of a child's parents are allergy sufferers, the child is more likely to develop the condition.

> However, other factors come into play too, because some people with two allergic parents never suffer from the condition themselves.
> One of the most important of these factors is the ability to combat stress. The better you can handle

Our emotions and the immune system

Our immune system has a very close and permanent relationship with our emotions. This relationship is maintained with the aid of certain neuro-hormones, which are produced by the brain when it experiences pressure and danger. These hormones circulate within the body and make contact with receptors on the surface of the white corpuscles. Our moods and feelings therefore have a direct influence on the responses of the immune system. So it could be that a violent argument directly contributes to the onset of a cough or to the reappearance of a cold sore.

Similarly, some people believe that allergic responses are sometimes triggered by strong emotions and that stress can cause the onset of asthma attacks and other reactions.

Avoid conflict and harmful relationships

People with allergies need to protect themselves from stress. Avoid conflict: learn to back down when the cause of the argument isn't important. Say what you think, but never aggressively: keeping your feelings bottled up results in enormous stress, but explosions of anger usually only make matters worse. Always make time for things you enjoy: go for a walk, see a movie, go on holiday.

nervous tension and your emotions, the more likely you are to avoid asthma and other allergies, even if you are genetically predisposed to suffer from the condition.

KEY FACTS

* Stress exacerbates all allergies, especially asthma.

* This occurs because there is a close and permanent relationship between the brain and the immune system.

* The better you are able to handle stress and to control your emotions, the better you will manage your episodes of asthma.

34 learn to relax

Daily stress can be combated by developing your own regime of relaxation. There are many different techniques to help you to relax.

Techniques that focus on the physical Some techniques concentrate on relaxing the body first in order to induce a state of mental serenity. This is the basic principle of Schultz's autogenic training: you lie down, breathe deeply and try to imagine the physical sensations of warmth, heaviness and then coolness. Subsequently, the mere act of thinking about the experience will immediately induce a state of complete physical and mental relaxation, regardless of the circumstances.

Techniques that concentrate on the mind Other techniques, such as sophrology and visualization, put the emphasis on first relaxing the mind. At the beginning of the session, a little time is devoted to physical relaxation (deep breathing, relaxing the muscles, etc.) but the rest of the session concentrates exclusively on visualizing relaxing and soothing scenarios. The closer the images are to reality, the greater their effect will be.

●●● D I D   Y O U   K N O W ?

> Breathing is always a central feature of relaxation techniques.
> It is the only vital function that involves both body and mind, which is why it is used as the quickest way of reaching a state of complete relaxation.

K E Y   F A C T S

∗ Relaxation techniques are effective ways of handling stress.

∗ Try autogenic training, sophrology or visualization.

35 eat quail's eggs

These delightful little birds lay eggs that appear to offer particular benefits for allergy sufferers. Their eggs may be small and fragile, but they may offer relief to some sufferers.

A surprise in the sixties In 1967 the wife of a quail breeder realized that, for no apparent reason, the asthma attacks which had affected her for many years had suddenly disappeared. Then one of the farm workers noticed the same thing had happened to him. The quail breeder distributed eggs to allergy sufferers in the neighbourhood, and they all seemed to be cured, too. Since then, over 200 studies have confirmed that the quail breeder's hunch was right.

An enemy of immunoglobulins The effectiveness of quail's eggs is attributed to the fact that they curb the production of immunoglobulins and ease inflammation. They can prevent as well as cure: if you suffer from seasonal allergies, start treatment two months before the symptoms begin; if your allergies occur all year round, take a course on a regular basis, say one month out of every three.

● ● ● DID YOU KNOW?

> The prescribed dose is six eggs a day: not exactly a diet that can be sustained over a long period of time. However, health-food shops now stock food supplements that contain a base of quail's eggs.

KEY FACTS

* Quail's eggs curb the production of immunoglobulins and reduce the responses of the immune system.

* They also have an anti-inflammatory effect.

* They can be taken in the form of food supplements.

Yoga reduces stress and improves the functioning of the immune system. So it's very good for allergy sufferers, if they choose the right positions to practise.

36

adopt the fish position

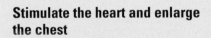

Stimulate the heart and enlarge the chest

The ancient discipline of yoga brings together body and mind in harmony. It helps you to eliminate tension and lets you handle your emotions better. People suffering from respiratory allergies ought to practise it for these reasons alone, but, in addition, some positions have a direct effect on your breathing. This is particularly true of the fish position. Practised regularly, it stimulates blood circulation, is good for the skin and, above all, enlarges the chest, so improving breathing.

The fish

❶ Lie flat on your back on the ground with your legs stretched, toes pointed, arms wide open in the form of a cross. Hollow your back to lift it off the ground so you are resting on your buttocks and the top of your skull. Stretch out your neck as far as you can. Hold this position for three seconds while continuing to breathe regularly.

❷ Without changing your back's position, put your hands together above your chest (as if you were praying) and lift your left leg without lifting your hip from the ground. Hold this position for three seconds.

❸ Lower the left leg and, bringing your arms down to your sides, slide your palms under your back, supporting your weight on your elbows. Hold for three seconds.

❹ Lift the right leg, while stretching out your arms, keeping your hands together. Hold the position for three seconds. Lower your arms and leg, then relax for twenty seconds before starting again.

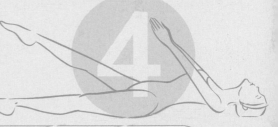

KEY FACTS

∗ Yoga brings body and mind into harmony and calms stress and emotions.

∗ Some positions have a direct effect upon the respiratory system.

∗ This is particularly true of the fish position, which strengthens the heart and enlarges the chest, thus improving breathing.

37

consult a psycho-therapist

Everyone has used the expression 'it took my breath away'. When we experience powerful emotions, we literally do become breathless. This is just one example of the close link between breathing and our feelings.

Breathless

We are psychosomatic creatures: our thoughts and feelings have a close, intricate relationship with the functions of our body. Breathing is the key link between these two elements of our being. It is the only vital function that is both voluntary and involuntary: we can control our breathing, speed it up, even stop it (until we start to suffocate); but we continue to breathe when we are

●●● DID YOU KNOW?

> Marcel Proust was famously asthmatic. A sickly child at a time when there were few effective treatments, he was totally dominated by the strong personality of his mother.
> The mother–child relationship has a big influence on child development, especially in the context of chronic ill health. When this

relationship becomes too intense, and if the father is absent, the child has trouble separating his inner self and the external world.
> Proust was 'invaded' by his environment and could not defend himself against it, just as he was 'invaded' by

asleep and sometimes we lose control of it when we hyperventilate. That is why breathing is the first vital function to be disturbed when we experience violent emotions.

What is taking your breath away?

Respiratory problems, particularly hyperventilation, are sometimes directly caused by a psychological problem – some emotional disturbance that has physical repercussions. In such cases, you should see a psychotherapist to resolve the problem.

Some therapies only involve discussion, while others also work on 'the memory of the body'. Of course, not all respiratory allergies have a psychological origin, but it might be worthwhile exploring the possibility.

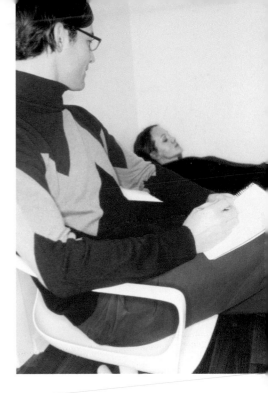

the presence of his mother. He remained dependent on her all his life. He was so asthmatic that he suffered attacks merely by looking at Van Gogh's *Sunflowers* painting!

> There is a strong possibility that his asthma was caused, or certainly exacerbated, by this complex family dynamic and psychological disturbance.

 KEY FACTS

* Breathing is a physical function that is closely linked with the emotions.

* Sometimes respiratory symptoms are the result of past psychological traumas.

* Psychotherapy can help to solve the problem.

38

vitamins can help

Certain vitamins help to ensure that the immune system does not overreact. A well-chosen programme of vitamins provides a very good defence against such attacks.

Amazing vitamin C

A good supply of vitamin C improves the working of the whole immune system, including its response to allergens. There is some evidence to suggest that regular doses of this vitamin will reduce both the frequency and severity of asthma and hay fever attacks. Preferably, choose a natural vitamin C with a base of cynorodon or acerola. This is easily

●●● DID YOU KNOW?

> Among the B group vitamins, B5 is the most useful for treating allergies. It is found in large quantities in royal jelly, the substance made by bees to feed the queen of the hive.
> Royal jelly contains eight essential amino acids and numerous vitamins and trace elements, as well as the important neurotransmitter acetylcholine. Such exceptional richness makes it a super-food. Allergy sufferers could benefit from taking regular three-week courses of this natural food supplement several times a year.

assimilated by the body and does not cause either nervous irritation or digestive problems. The recommended daily dosage is quite small: 60mg per day for an adult. However, larger amounts can be taken to combat tiredness, stress and pollution but only under the guidance of your doctor. Remember, though, that too much vitamin C can be harmful.

Some B group vitamins

The B group vitamins, especially B5, B6 and B12, are also useful weapons in the war against allergies. They are mainly found in wholemeal cereals (such as bread and pasta), fish, pulses, liver and egg yolk. You could, from time to time, take a course of B vitamins or eat some brewer's yeast.

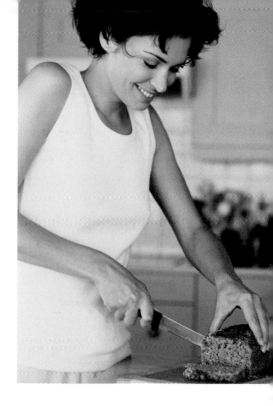

> Royal jelly is available in health-food shops in various forms, such as small bottle doses, phials and capsules. It is sold by itself or combined with other substances, such as ginseng. The recommended dosage varies according to the form in which it is sold.

KEY FACTS

* Regular doses of natural vitamin C can reduce both the frequency and severity of asthma and hay fever attacks.

* B group vitamins, especially B5, are thought to help fight allergies.

39

supplement your trace elements

These micronutrients, particularly copper and manganese, which are present in the body in tiny quantities, affect the functioning of the immune system and its susceptibility to allergies. You should take regular supplements of them, but don't overdo it.

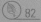

Manganese: the best trace element for allergies

Manganese is a genuine anti-allergy mineral and has an effect on all reactions, however severe. Humans seldom suffer from a lack of manganese, but research has shown that maintaining a high level of the substance in the body is an effective treatment for hay fever and allergic asthma, as well as for skin allergies such as eczema and nettle rash.

Manganese is found in large quantities in almonds, pecans, walnuts and tea, but not in many other foods. This makes it difficult to eat some at every meal, of course, so the most convenient way to consume it is in supplement form, available from pharmacies. (Most general multivitamin supplements also contain a reasonable amount of manganese.)

Copper, sulphur, cobalt

To treat all allergies, you can combine manganese with sulphur, which makes a wonderful natural desensitizer. Other combinations of trace elements provide more specific treatments:

- manganese and cobalt effecti... relieve hay fever symptoms;
- manganese and copper are good for asthma sufferers, especially those who also suffer from bronchitis.

A healthy diet

However, you should remember that it is usually preferable to have a good, mixed diet that covers all the major food groups, but, failing that, your doctor or pharmacy will be able to advise you about supplements.

Visits to spas and health resorts have been recommended for centuries as treatments for respiratory problems, including those caused by allergies. These are the places to go for pure air and water rich in minerals.

Treating asthma Water rich in bicarbonates is effective in the relief of bronchial spasms and reduces the production of histamine. Some resorts specialize in treating asthmatic children. High-altitude health resorts are also recommended: the altitude and dry, cold air offer respite for people suffering as a result of house-dust mites in their own homes.

Treating hay fever Hay fever sufferers also benefit from taking the waters. As for asthmatics, bicarbonate water is recommended, while sulphurated water can help cure chronic hay fever. Sulphur also relieves inflammation in the mucous membranes and the lungs.

● ● ● DID YOU KNOW?

> A water cure can help combat allergies.

> Breathing pure air has obvious, considerable benefits.

> All the major spas now have sites on the Internet, where you will be able to learn if they offer treatments appropriate to you.

KEY FACTS

* Taking the waters is a very good way of treating asthma and hay fever.

* Bicarbonate and sulphurated waters are most frequently prescribed.

case study

It took me two years to get rid of my asthma

« I had my first asthma attacks when I was five or six years old. My parents discovered what I was allergic to and made sure I didn't come into contact with it any more. There were no problems for a few weeks, but then it all started up again, because I'd become allergic to something else. The same process continued throughout my childhood. Eventually, I thought I could deal with it, but do you ever really get used to that kind of pain? When I got married, my wife, who's interested in natural forms of medicine, encouraged me to take a different approach to my illness. She took charge of everything: what I ate, courses of vitamins and minerals, relaxation and so on. I started to take physical exercise again, not having done any for years. I was already feeling much better, but it was a homeopathic doctor who finally got rid of my asthma. It took a long time, nearly two years, to overcome it completely. I followed a basic course of treatment regularly and a special crisis course when my symptoms worsened. Now I lead a normal life. »

41 >>>

>> **Your skin reddens, it itches,** you scratch it, sometimes it bleeds. It seems to heal, but then suddenly flares up again. Eczema is a real nightmare. It affects people of all ages, including babies, and can become chronic.

>>>> **You must find the allergen that is responsible.** Often, once you have located it, you must avoid all contact with it if the problem is to be cured permanently.

>>>>> **If that doesn't work,** there are water cures, vitamins, relaxation, homeopathy and herbs to help you.

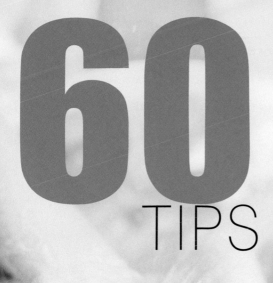

60
TIPS

41

what exactly is the problem?

Skin allergies can take various forms, ranging from common nettle rash (urticaria) at one extreme to the very dangerous angioneurotic oedema at the other, with stubborn eczema somewhere in the middle. Before starting a treatment, you need to identify your problem precisely.

What have you touched?

The most common skin allergy is contact dermatitis. It is caused by direct contact with allergenic substances, which penetrate the skin. Once the allergens are recognized as 'invaders', a reaction occurs around the place of contact. It takes a few hours for the first signs to appear, and sometimes a day or so before the symptoms develop fully. The skin becomes red and itchy, and may swell and exhibit tiny blisters. Itching leads to scratching, then

●●● DID YOU KNOW?

> The most effective course of action is to avoid all contact with the allergen, but first you need to identify it.
> The area affected should provide the first clue: if it's on your hands, the culprit could be a product you have touched or your ring; if it's on your face, you might need to change your cream or make-up remover; if it's on your body, it could be due to your clothes, your washing powder or your perfume.
> Allergies occuring on the ear lobes are easy: they are nearly always caused by earrings containing nickel.

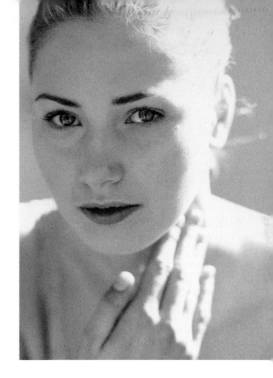

to infection with weeping, oozy skin. Often the source of the rash is obvious – a red, circluar lesion under your wrist-watch or the rash on your neck after you have applied perfume – but sometimes the problem is harder to pinpoint.

Other types of eczema include atopic, which is common and runs in families, occuring in small children. Detergents and strong chemicals can cause an irritant dermatitis, especially common in hair-dressers or bar staff. Irritant dermatitis makes allergic contact dermatitis more likely; while people with atopic eczema are more prone to irritant dermatitis.

Nettle rash or eczema?

In cases of nettle rash (urticaria), red, raised marks appear on the skin, similar to those caused by stinging nettles, and are very itchy. The symptoms appear and disappear quickly – usually over hours; the surface of the skin is unchanged and there is no scarring. Its triggers include many drugs (antibiotics, painkillers, seda-tives, diuretics), some foodstuffs (nuts, fish, eggs, chocolate) and even the envi-ronment (air pressure, cold, light, heat).

Eczema causes areas of the skin to red-den and start to itch while becoming weepy, then dry and cracked. Unlike nettle rash, it often also becomes infected. It affects mainly children.

 KEY FACTS

* Contact dermatitis causes red marks and itching.

* Nettle rash develops quickly. It might be due to substance intolerance rather than a genuine allergy.

* Eczema causes the skin to weep, then become dry and cracked.

42

try a detox programme

One of the main ways in which the body excretes toxins is through the skin. However, when it is also affected by allergies, the skin needs some help. Try treating it to a regular detox programme, such as one involving fresh juice.

Help your skin to cleanse the body

The body's many metabolic activities generate large amounts of waste, such as urea, uric acid and dead cells. These toxins are removed by the excretory organs: the liver, kidneys, lungs, and, just as crucially, the skin. It's a good idea for people who suffer from skin allergies to try a detox cure two or three times a year to give the skin some respite.

●●● DID YOU KNOW?

> If you invest in a juice extractor, you will be able to prepare a wide variety of juices, and many more than are available in the supermarket (for example, cress, chicory, celery, sweet potatoes, melon).

> Always wash fruit and vegetables (but not for too long) and then lightly peel them.
> Cut them into little pieces after you have removed their stones or seeds.

You could get into the habit of introducing fresh fruit or vegetable juices into your daily diet, at breakfast time, for example, or as an aperitif, instead of alcohol. You could also try a juice detox programme.

A three-day programme

To do this, start by gradually eliminating protein (meat, fish, eggs and so on) from your meals, then do the same with all animal fats (butter, cheese) and finally with oils and cereals. This preparatory phase should last a week.
When you are eating just fruit and vegetables, the next stage is a liquid-only diet of fruit and vegetable juices (as much as you like) for three days. Choose those that you can digest easily and that don't cause you stomach acidity or bloating. After the three days, return gradually to your normal diet. The best times to carry out this programme are when the seasons are changing.

> Press fruit and vegetables separately. When mixing the juices, start with the thickest ones.
> Drink the juice as soon as it is ready.

KEY FACTS

* The skin is one of the organs that remove toxins resulting from cellular metabolism.

* If you suffer from skin allergies, it's a good idea to make this task easier for your skin.

* Fresh fruit and vegetable juices help the body to excrete toxins and simultaneously provide it with plenty of vitamins and minerals.

43 clean out your intestines

The intestines form a major part of the body's excretory system, but, in addition to eliminating waste, they play an important role in the human immune system. It's not surprising, then, that they affect allergies. They will work better if you give them a little help.

● ● ● DID YOU KNOW?

> Exponents of natural medicine place great importance on their patients' intestines functioning well, which is why they advocate enemas.

> Some even favour a more forceful technique, namely colonic irrigation. This is a modern, more elaborate kind of 'super enema'. It is carried out by a trained therapist. You will need at least three sessions for the therapy to have an effect.

Putting the emphasis on defence

Elimination of waste matter is not the only function of the intestines. They are also involved in the digestion and absorption of food, and in the body's immune defences. The bacteria that live in them play an essential role in these defences: they line the intestinal walls and prevent certain toxins from penetrating into the bloodstream, while allowing essential nutrients to pass through. These bacteria kill fungi, viruses and harmful bacteria. They are also involved in the elimination of dead cells and free radicals, which our metabolism produces continuously and which must be removed.

Obviously, if your intestines are in a poor condition, they will play a less effective role as part of your immune system, thus increasing the risk of allergies among susceptible people.

Leeks, prunes, mallow and marsh mallow

There are certain vegetables, fruits and plants that you can eat to help your intestines perform all their functions. First, eat leeks regularly. They are composed of long fibres made of cellulose and mucilage, which clean out accumulated impurities rather like a brush. You might also try prunes and dried figs, which act in the same way, and, in addition, have a slight laxative effect.

If you suffer from sluggish intestines, give them some help. Chronic constipation contributes to skin problems in general and skin allergies in particular. From time to time, drink herbal teas made from slightly laxative, soothing plants such as mallow and marsh mallow. They are a natural, gentle way of helping your intestines do their work.

> Then the intestines will then need to be replenished with 'good' bacteria.

KEY FACTS

* The intestines play an essential role in our immune defences.

* When they function poorly, these defences are weakened, which increases the risk of allergic reactions.

* To help them, eat leeks, prunes or dried figs, and drink herbal teas.

44

regenerate your intestinal flora

Not all bacteria are harmful. Some, like those found inside our intestines, are good for us. Without them, our immune system would suffer, so pamper them a little. You will be glad you did.

Billions of faithful friends

There are billions of good bacteria nestling in the nooks and crannies of our intestines, where they reproduce. They are our good friends, but sometimes we destroy huge numbers of them with our bad eating habits, stress, antibiotics and in many other ways. Obviously this should be avoided, but it is also important to maintain a balance between the various types of bacteria. For example,

Candida albicans is naturally present in the digestive system, where it has a vital role to play, but sometimes stress or poor diet allows it to multiply much more quickly than the other digestive bacteria. It then relocates to areas of the body where it has no right to be and causes some unpleasant symptoms, especially on the skin. If you suffer from skin allergies, you should make an effort to avoid such imbalances.

Yoghurts and whey

To reproduce successfully, 'good' intestinal bacteria need nourishment and the introduction of new strains. There are products on the market that meet both needs, since they contain sugars especially suitable for the bacteria and yeasts rich in bacterial strains. If you follow a special diet of these products two or three times a year, you will keep your intestinal flora in good condition. You could also regularly eat yoghurt containing plenty of bifidobacteria, which reinforce the 'good' bacteria already in the gut. Whey, the yellowish liquid you often find on the surface of yoghurts, has the same effect. It contains bacteria produced during milk fermentation. It can be consumed fresh or in granule or capsule form.

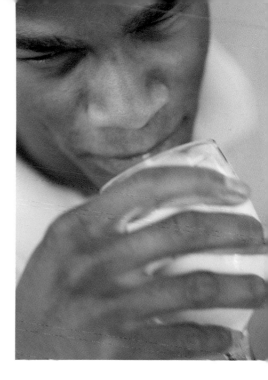

 KEY FACTS

* We need a large, well-balanced population of 'good' bacteria in our intestines to avoid certain skin complaints.

* Eating yoghurt and whey will help to provide this.

* Also eat food supplements enriched with yeast.

45

be careful in the sun

You can't wait for your holiday to arrive and when it does, you find yourself covered in red blotches, itchy rashes and prickly heat. You are allergic to the sun. This situation has to be dealt with if you are going to enjoy being near the sea at the height of the summer.

Sun allergies

The sun is vital for life to flourish but contact with just a few of its powerful rays can sometimes cause an allergic reaction in the skin. These sun or heat rashes can mean that on the first day of your holidays you break out in red, itchy blotches. In order to prevent this from happening you need to take the following precautions:

• Never go out in the sun during the hottest times of the day, ie between 11 am and 5 pm.

• Make sure you supply your skin with all the necessary nutrients – vitamins A and C (see Tip 54) and vegetable oils (see Tip 53).

• Wear a protective suncream and make sure you look closely at its ingredients. Avoid creams containing perfume and bergamot.

Try homeopathy

Homeopathic remedies can be an effective protection against sun allergies. There is one important remedy that can help most conditions: *Muriaticum acidum* taken in a dosage of 15C once a week during the month prior to exposure can prevent symptoms occurring. Taken in the form of granules (dosage 7C, taken 3 times a day), it is the best treatment to take once the symptoms have appeared. Depending on your own individual needs, it is possible to take the granules in conjunction with other medications.

• If you suffer from extremely itchy skin, take *Urica uren* (7C), in particular if the condition is made worse by contact with water and the cold.

• If the itchiness is not accompanied by either redness or an eruption of the skin, try *Dolichos pluriens* 7C.

• If the itchiness is aggravated by heat and improved by the cold, take *Apis mellifica* 7C.

● ● ●   DID YOU KNOW?

> In most cases, a sun allergy is the result of interaction between a sensitising substance and the sun's rays. Some medications can form the basis of this allergy, such as antibiotics, quinine derivatives, some anti-depressants or anti-inflammatory drugs.

> Substances that are contained in perfumes and other cosmetics can also trigger a reaction, even if there is no reaction when not exposed to the sun.

> Sometimes, the combination of the sun and iodine (at the seaside) or sun and pollen (in the countryside) can be the culprit.

KEY FACTS

∗ An allergy to the sun is generally due to two factors: a sensitising agent and the rays of the sun.

∗ In order to prevent such an allergy, avoid going out in the sun during the hottest time of the day and make sure you protect your skin properly.

∗ Try homeopathic remedies.

46 take care when gardening

If you have a garden, as well as protecting yourself from the sun, you need to look out for insects and chemicals. Fertilizers, fungicides and pesticides can sometimes irritate your skin.

Plants that make you itch Of course, you need to be careful about insects (see Tip 5) when you are in the garden, but there are other, less obvious, dangers, too. Some plants are irritants, or even poisonous. Everyone knows the damage that stinging nettles can do, but not as many people are aware that the seemingly innocent primrose can cause similar reactions. The same is true of sumach (poison ivy), mango and *Ginkgo biloba*, among many others.

Products that make you scratch Today's gardeners are offered a huge range of products to help them beat the insects and make their roses bloom, but many of them are potential irritants. Avoid using chemical fertilizers and pesticides and opt for traditional, natural methods instead. Nettle or comfrey slurry, for example, is an excellent plant food. To make it, just soak nettles or comfrey in a tightly sealed bucket of water for about a month.

KEY FACTS

* When gardening, be careful of insects and the sun, but also of plants that irritate or sting and chemical-rich gardening products.

* Choose the organic approach instead: nettle slurry, compost and ladybirds to eat aphids.

47 spring water to the rescue

A water cure is a very effective way of treating skin complaints, particularly eczema. Products with a base of spring water are also available.

Resorts that specialize Some spa resorts specialize in treating skin problems. Their waters are very rich in trace elements and have a level of acidity (similar to the skin's), which means they don't harm the beneficial bacteria on the skin's surface. Spa waters therefore soothe without causing any harm. Each spa has water with unique properties, so choose the one that is best for you.

Products that work Some resorts have developed ranges of cosmetics, with a base of spring water, which have all the therapeutic qualities you would expect. Each product contains a large quantity of spring water (about 80 per cent) and all the other constituents are selected on the basis that they are very unlikely to cause an allergic reaction. If you invariably suffer a reaction with conventional skin-care products, they might be the answer.

● ● ● DID YOU KNOW?

> Try spraying yourself with mineral water. The tiny droplets safely cleanse the skin and don't have any of the disadvantages of tap water. What's more, the trace elements found in spring water are absorbed by the skin.

KEY FACTS

* Some spa resorts are amazingly successful with the treatment of skin allergies, especially eczema.

* They have developed ranges of cosmetics with a base of spring water that are also very effective.

48 wash yourself naturally

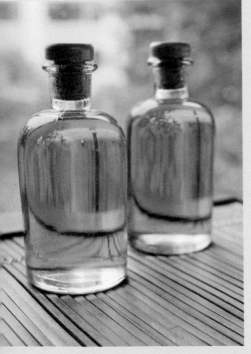

Do you love foam baths and perfumed soap? Well, if you have skin problems, you might have to do without them, as they often cause allergies. In addition, the detergents they contain degrease the skin and make it more sensitive to potential allergens. Choose products which contain no soap or detergent.

● ● ● DID YOU KNOW?

> If your skin is very sensitive, it might react to some essential oils. Therefore, prepare your mixture of oils and test a drop of it on the inside of your wrist. Wait for a quarter of an hour. If no red mark appears, go ahead and put it in your bathwater.

> Choose 100 per cent pure and natural, preferably organic, essential

Now wash your hands...

Doctors are rediscovering the value of elementary hygiene, and particularly of washing your hands. This simple act on its own is enough to limit the spread of many infections. However, you need to be careful about the products you use, because many of the bars of soap currently available contain allergenic substances such as lanolin and glycerine. The cleansing agents they contain are often 'aggressive' and make the skin more sensitive.

It is much better to use soap-free cleansing bars: they have a similar level of acidity to that of the skin and do it no harm. You might miss the luxuriant foam, but they clean you just as well, with much less risk. You can also buy liquid soap-free cleansers. Most soap-free products contain no perfume, so the risk of an allergic reaction is further reduced. Detergents can also damage the skin, so use emollients such as aqueous cream instead.

oils. Oils that make no such claims are sometimes synthetic or semi-synthetic. These oils lack the good qualities of the pure ones, and could even be allergenic themselves.

... and then wash all over

Most bath foams and shower gels also contain 'aggressive' cleaning agents that make the skin more vulnerable to allergenic substances, particularly those found in synthetic perfumes. If you adore lazing in the bath, try using essential oils instead. First, wash yourself with soap-free cleanser, then run yourself a 'pleasure bath'. Put a dozen or so drops of soothing essential oils on to a tablespoon and hold it under a fast-running tap. Among the most relaxing oils are lavender, camomile and rosewood.

KEY FACTS

* The most commonly used soaps and bath foams are both 'aggressive' and allergenic.

* Choose soap-free cleansing bars or liquids.

* Never use bubble bath.

* Use essential oils like lavender, neroli and rosewood to add an extra element of relaxation to your bath.

49

choose your cosmetics with care

Applying and removing make-up and general skin care are not simple matters for women whose skin is affected by allergies. Fortunately, there are products available nowadays that are specially designed for sensitive skins.

Do your own market research

Almost all cosmetics contain some potentially allergenic substances. However, just because you are allergic to one product, doesn't mean you'll be allergic to all of them. If you suffer a reaction, first identify the product responsible, then try other brands, carefully reading the labels to ensure that they don't contain the same ingredients as the one that caused the problem. If you can't work out what is causing your reaction,

●●● DID YOU KNOW?

> You need to take great care over the use of perfumes and deodorants. Both can cause violent reactions.

> Instead of a deodorant, why not use an alum stone? It closes the pores and naturally reduces the effects of perspiration without leaving an odour.

> Nowadays, almost all perfumes, even the most well-known brands, contain potentially allergenic synthetic essences.

your doctor might suggest special skin tests (known as patch testing) to identify the culprit. As a general rule, the more complex the composition of a product, the greater the risk of it containing an allergenic substance. So trust in simplicity or go for products specially designed to avoid all allergic reactions (often labelled 'dermatologically tested').

Cosmetics, the gentle, natural way

The simplest products to use when removing make-up are a bar of soap-free cleanser and a mineral-water spray. They are effective and harmless. As far as creams are concerned, choose those that contain spring water (see Tip 47). They soothe irritations and are specially designed for very sensitive skin.

If you want to make yourself a face mask, try using natural clay. Prepare a paste made of clay, mineral water and three drops of essential oil (lavender or neroli). Spread it on your face and keep it there for about a quarter of an hour. Then wash it off with mineral water.

As far as make-up is concerned, there are no miracle solutions, as almost all make-up products contain preservatives, solar filters or colouring agents capable of causing reactions. Try to stick to cosmetics whose contents are as natural as possible.

> If your favourite perfume triggers allergic reactions, there is only one solution: stop wearing it!

KEY FACTS

* Not all cosmetics contain the same ingredients. Test a variety until you come across those that are best for you.

* Consider natural alternatives: use clay for face masks and alum stone instead of a deodorant.

103

50

renew your wardrobe

If your skin is very sensitive, be sure to wear the right clothes. Some materials are very allergenic. Choose natural textiles: rediscover the pleasures of hemp, linen and cotton.

The relationship between skin and fabrics

Many cases of contact dermatitis are caused by our clothes. The fabrics we wear and our skin exchange molecules and ions, so they need to get along. Many people seem to have adverse reactions to synthetic fibres, especially polyester. Read the labels carefully, and, where possible, choose natural fibres such as cotton, linen, silk and hemp.

●●● DID YOU KNOW?

> Clothes have been made out of natural fibres, such as linen, hemp and cotton, for centuries.

> Artificial fibres are extracted from natural plant cells (usually from their cellulose), among them viscose and acetate.

> Synthetic fibres, such as acrylics, polyamides and elastane, are entirely man-made and are the most likely to cause allergic reactions.

Each natural fibre has its advantages

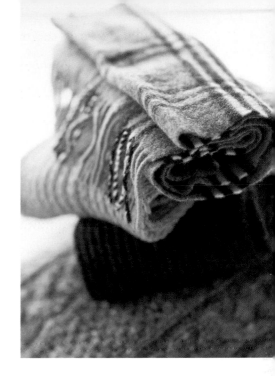

Cotton is not damaged by washing, although it does shrink; and is not allergenic, unless it has undergone excessive chemical treatment. It is best to choose clothes made of organic cotton, which is sure to be natural and untreated.

Nothing is better than wool for keeping you warm. It also lets your skin breathe and won't make it dry. It is a very safe material, and does not burn below 600°C (1,112°F), unlike most synthetic fibres. Its sole disadvantage is that people with eczema may react to it.

Linen is comfortable and cool and as such has a natural anti-stress effect.

Plant extracts are generally used for dyeing organic textiles. Not only do these dyes cause no allergic reactions but, in addition to their colours, they transfer some of their therapeutic qualities to the textiles. The plants that are used for orange dyes, for example, contain flavonoids, which protect the skin from fungi and mould.

KEY FACTS

* Synthetic and artificial fabrics often cause allergic reactions.

* To avoid them, choose natural fabrics such as cotton, silk, linen and wool.

* As far as possible, choose organically produced materials: their dyes are natural and can have therapeutic qualities.

51

the benefits of serenity

The skin and the brain are very closely linked. They communicate by means of chemical messengers. So it is unsurprising that the mind and emotions influence the way the skin reacts. Relaxation techniques can therefore soothe skin reactions.

Skin, mind and nervous system

The skin does much more than merely cover the body and protect it from external attacks. It is an organ in its own right, involved in numerous vital activities, such as breathing, excretion and sensory perception.

● ● ● DID YOU KNOW?

> Throughout the ages, people have used their skin as a message board. In traditional societies, marks on the skin indicated social rank or religious belief.

> Modern tattoos are usually less symbolic, but they still express identity.

> However, if you have sensitive skin and are subject to allergic reactions, tattoos and piercings are not good ideas. They constitute an 'attack' on the skin, even when carried out in professional, hygienic conditions.

The skin is the mirror of the soul

This is not a new idea, but recently it has been confirmed by science. Skin problems are caused by a great many factors (allergic, genetic, environmental) but their psychological dimension can no longer be ignored. Studies show that the skin is in constant, complex communication with the brain and the nervous system.

A healthy mind in a healthy skin

An allergic reaction might be your skin's way of telling you that you should be more relaxed. The more serene, calm and at peace with yourself you are, the better equipped your skin will be to carry out its various functions. Relaxation will help you to deal with your allergies (see Tip 34). Choose the technique that suits you best and fits most neatly into your daily life.

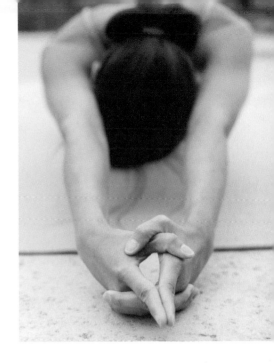

> Body piercings and tattooing might transmit blood-borne viruses, such as hepatitis, or lead to skin infections. You might also become allergic to the dyes in the tattoo or the metals in the piercing stud.

KEY FACTS

* Recent scientific studies have confirmed what people have known intuitively for thousands of years: the skin is the mirror of the soul.

* Skin problems very often have a psychological dimension, to a greater or lesser extent.

* Relax: calmness and serenity will do your skin good.

52 treat yourself to floral elixirs

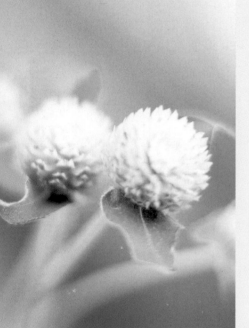

Flowers soothe us: when we see them, smell them or touch them. You might not know it, but they can be even more soothing if you drink them. Floral elixirs, developed in the early twentieth century by Dr Edward Bach, can control the intense emotions that sometimes leave their marks on sensitive skins.

●●● DID YOU KNOW?

> Several of the elixirs are suited to the sensitive personalities of allergy sufferers.

> Nutmeg calms the fear that something dreadful (but unspecific) is about to happen. Such fear is psychologically destructive and makes the skin highly sensitive.

> Busy Lizzie soothes irritable, edgy people whose skin reddens at the slightest upset.

An unexpected recovery

Dr Bach lived in England in the early 1900s. He was diagnosed with cancer, and his medical colleagues gave him only a few months to live. But rather than resigning himself to the 'inevitable', he continued working. World War I had just broken out and he thought that he could be useful.

Three months later, Edward Bach was in full remission. He attributed his cure to his powerful motivation, to his profound desire to live in order to help other people. It had become clear to him that mental attitude was a crucial factor in the process of recovery from illness, and that all illnesses emerged from an emotional and mental disturbance.

From a love of nature

Having devised this theory, he began to look for natural remedies that could regulate people's moods and feelings. He closed his consulting room and took walks in the English countryside. While there, he realized that 'All of the plant's power to cure is concentrated in its flower.' So he collected morning dew lying on flower petals and administered it to patients. He obtained some encouraging results. Gradually he discovered correspondences between our different states of mind and the dew from various flowers. He also developed a procedure for harnessing the power of flowers and turning it into a remedy. The thirty-eight Bach elixirs were created. Others later built upon Dr Bach's work and produced their own elixirs from flowers growing in various parts of the world, such as the Alps, Australia and California.

These elixirs can be bought in the form of drops in pharmacies that specialize in herbal medicine, and in health-food shops. The drops are taken in courses that last for three weeks or more.

> Clematis helps bring dreamers back to reality and helps them appreciate the good points of the world around them, even when their skin is annoying them.

KEY FACTS

* Floral elixirs were created by an English doctor, Edward Bach.

* They calm and control intense emotions.

* You can take courses of them in the form of drops, which are available in some pharmacies and in health-food shops.

53 the benefits of raw plant oils

To be healthy, our skin needs numerous nutrients, particularly essential fatty acids, and a healthy skin is more resistant to allergies.

When skin cells lack lipids The membrane of skin cells is mainly made up of lipids. If there are not enough lipids in this membrane, it hardens and the exchanges between cells deteriorate. The skin becomes dry, red, sensitive, fragile and susceptible to various disorders. A skin well nourished by essential fatty acids, on the other hand, is in a much better position to resist disorders, including allergic ones.

It takes some time, but it's worth it You therefore need to consume raw plant oils, since they contain the most vital essential fatty acids. Evening primrose oil and borage oil are particularly recommended. They are available in capsule form in health-food shops and pharmacies (take four to six per day). It will be at least six weeks before you see any improvement, but when it finally comes, it should last.

KEY FACTS

* Skin cells need essential fatty acids in order to function properly.

* Consume raw plant oils, especially evening primrose oil and borage oil.

54 essential supplements for your skin

The skin consumes many vitamins and minerals. If you do not keep it well supplied, the result could be skin allergies. It might be time to start taking supplements.

Vitamins that are good for the skin
People susceptible to skin allergies should take regular courses of vitamin supplements to keep their skin in good condition. Vitamins A, C and E are all vital for the skin, because they are powerful antioxidants and protect it from the ravages of free radicals. The B vitamins, especially B2 and B8, help to combat eczema.

Minerals that are good for the skin The skin needs copper and iron, but you must never exceed the prescribed dose of either. Copper is a particularly good treatment for infected eczema. Zinc is important for wound healing. Don't forget to take manganese and sulphur – the two trace elements that are most helpful for all allergy sufferers (see Tip 39).

.

●●● DID YOU KNOW?

> If you have a normal balanced diet you should not really need to take supplements, but they may be necessary after illness, surgery and for people on strict diets.
> Iron makes the blood healthy – consequently it imparts a healthy pink glow to your skin.

KEY FACTS

∗ Your skin needs vitamins A, C and E (antioxidants) and B group vitamins (to combat eczema).

∗ As for minerals, take iron and copper supplements but only the prescribed amount.

55

homeopathic pills can help

In addition to basic treatments designed to reduce allergic reactions generally, homeopathy offers some that are specifically designed for skin complaints. As always with this form of medicine, a personal treatment plan is devised for each patient by the practitioner.

Eczema: where, when, how?

When treating eczema, a good homeopathic doctor will look for the answers to several questions. Where is it situated? When did it appear? How did it develop? An outbreak of eczema can be dry or wet, pink or white; it can cause thin or thick pieces of dead skin to flake off; it can be exacerbated by heat or cold, sunshine or water.

- If the eczema is pink and slightly swollen, you need to take Apis.
- If the condition worsens after exposure to sunshine or contact with sea water, take Natrum Muriaticum. If it is more severe in the cold of winter, choose Petroleum.
- If the affected skin crumbles to a fine dust, soothe the condition with Arsenicum Album, but if large pieces of dead skin flake off, Arsenicum Iodatum is the better option.

The location of the eczema is another factor affecting choice of remedy: around the mouth (Sepia); on the fold inside the elbow (Berberis Vulgaris); on the scalp (Oleander); behind the ears (Graphites).

Nettle rash: hot or cold?

Homeopathy can relieve outbreaks of nettle rash, too, provided the appropriate treatment is selected. If the rash is made worse by the cold and causes itching that is almost painful, try Urtica Urens, particularly if you also suffer from rheumatism.

If the affected areas are soothed by bathing in hot water, Arsenicum Album is what you need; but if the itching is calmed and the rash reduced by applications of cold water, choose Apis. If nettle rash is very common in your family,

Psorinum is likely to be effective. Finally, the choice of remedy will be different according to whether the outbreak is caused by milk (Dulcamara), meat (Antimonium Crudem), strawberries (Fragaria) or wine (Chloralum).

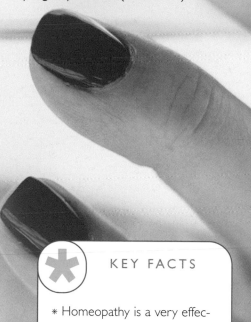

KEY FACTS

* Homeopathy is a very effective way of treating skin allergies.

* You should preferably consult a homeopathic doctor, who will be able to select the right remedy by taking all the key factors into account: location, cause, appearance and development.

56

Plants can be very good for your skin, especially if it is suffering from allergies. Some have soothing qualities, while others are moisturize or act as anti-inflammatories

put your trust in herbal medicine

Calendula – the best of the bunch

Calendula, the humble garden marigold, has beautiful yellow flowers that can work wonders healing and renewing damaged skin. They also soothe itching and are anti-inflammatory. The flowers contain beta-carotene, flavonoids, pectin and mucilages, so they also have nourishing, moisturizing and softening qualities. You can use *Calendula* as a mother-tincture and add it to your normal skin cream, or you can make your own lotion with it.

● ● ● DID YOU KNOW?

> Some plant oils have therapeutic effects on the skin. You can use them instead of a face cream or as a softening milk for the body.

> Select the oils according to the effect you want to achieve: evening primrose oil, borage oil and jojoba to nourish the skin (see Tip 53), apricot stone (to moisturize), St John's wort (anti-inflammatory) and wheatgerm (protective).

To make a lotion, gently boil 200g (7oz) of dried petals in 500ml (1 pint) of water for at least an hour, then filter carefully. Put some on your eczema or nettle rash every day. *Calendula* can also be taken internally: put a tablespoonful of dried petals into a large cup of boiling water and infuse for ten minutes. Drink up to three times a day. Do note that marigold should not be taken internally without first consulting a medical herbalist.

Infusions and poultices

Walnut tree leaves have been used to treat eczema for centuries. They are both an antiseptic (applied to the affected area) and a metabolic stimulant (taken internally). To make an infusion, put 10g ($^1/_3$oz) of leaves in 500ml (1pint) of boiling water and let them infuse for 10 minutes. Drink one cup in the morning and one in the evening.

Camomile is well known for its calming qualities. It also soothes burnt skin. Put 10 flowers in a bowl of boiling water and leave to infuse for 10 minutes.

You could also try cabbage poultices. At night, before going to bed, remove the big leaves from a cabbage, boil them for a few minutes, crush them carefully and then spread them over your skin, keeping them in place with gauze. It's a wonderful way to soothe eczema.

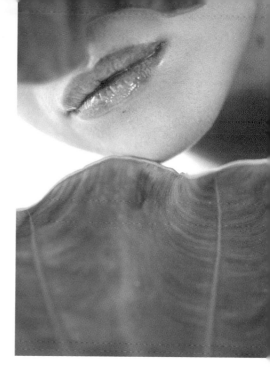

KEY FACTS

* Most skin problems can be treated effectively with plants.

* Calendula calms, soothes, heals and moisturizes.

* Some plants can be drunk as herbal teas and also used as poultices.

* Try using plant oils, such as apricot stone and St John's wort.

57

getting the point

Practitioners of Chinese medicine believe that skin problems are caused by disturbance in the flow of the body's energy. Conversely, the symptoms are relieved when a smooth flow is restored. If you locate the points you need to massage precisely, you should achieve rapid results.

A smooth flow

As with other allergies (see Tips 29 and 30), skin problems such as eczema and nettle rash can be relieved by practising jin shin do (*do-in*), a form of acupressure. Unlike acupuncture, no needles are used. Blocked energy will flow smoothly again when certain points on the body are stimulated with a finger. This form of massage must be done with precision, and quite forcefully. It also helps to relieve tension and negative emotions, such as anger and anxiety, to promote body-mind well-being.

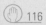

Hands and arms

If you have eczema, there are two points you can stimulate, one on the hand, the other on the arm. The first is on the back of the hand in the hollow between the thumb and the index finger. The other is in the fold of the elbow.

If you suffer from outbreaks of nettle rash, there are two points you should massage, although they are more difficult to locate. One is found just under the ankle bone on the inner side of the foot; the other is a little higher, two or three inches above the same bone.

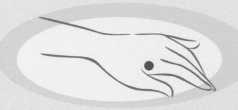
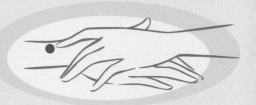

KEY FACTS

* Jin shin do (*do-in*) stimulates energy and rapidly relieves skin allergy symptoms.

* The massage points are found on the hands, arms and legs.

* You can practise jin shin do as soon as your symptoms occur or work out a programme that can be repeated every day over the course of several weeks.

58

finding your feet

Our feet are amazing. Not only do they get us from place to place; they cure our illnesses too, provided we massage them with loving care. Foot reflexology is both enjoyable and highly effective.

A map under our feet

The Chinese have drawn a map on the soles of the feet that represents the whole of the human body, including its internal organs. This is called a 'reflex zone'. Each of our organs corresponds with an area on the soles of the feet. When certain functions are hindered or harmed, the organ in question can be revived if you massage either the areas precisely corresponding to it or other areas that are linked to it in the energy flow network.

Taking your feet in hand

You can either go to a reflexology specialist or try it yourself at home. Massage
done by a specialist will be more precise
and therefore more effective, but it is
perfectly possible to massage yourself
and achieve good results.

Begin by massaging the whole of the foot
and ankle, preferably using plant oil (you
could also add a few drops of a soothing
essential oil, such as lavender or
camomile). Then concentrate on the
specific zones that are relevant to your
symptoms.

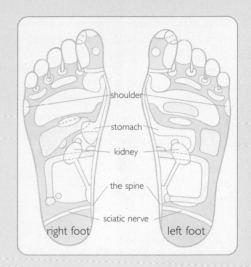

shoulder
stomach
kidney
the spine
sciatic nerve
right foot   left foot

KEY FACTS

* Our feet are 'reflex zones'. We can cure
many illnesses by massaging them.

* To cure allergies, concentrate on the zones
corresponding to the adrenal glands, the
kidneys, the bladder and the bronchial tubes.

* If a particular zone is painful at first,
don't worry. Keep massaging it and
the problem should ease.

59

don't be a shrinking violet

Expressions such as 'thick-skinned' and 'thin-skinned' suggest the connection between skin and personality. If you grow more confident, your skin will improve and reflect all the good qualities you possess inside. You could even say that you have 'saved your skin'!

Don't hide in the shadows

We all know unhappy teenagers who try to keep out of sight as much as possible. Obviously, the hormonal disturbances of adolescence go some way towards explaining their behaviour, but their spots and pimples also make them want to shrink away out of sight. The same applies to some adults who suffer from skin problems, especially when the eczema or nettle rash is on the face. But if you can manage to increase your self-confidence, go outside and meet other people, you will aid your skin's healing process.

Make a list of your good qualities

So, how can you enhance your self-confidence? Above all, by learning about yourself. Of course, it's not always easy to look fairly and kindly in the mirror, but some simple personal-development techniques will help you. For example, draw up a list of your good points and weaknesses. At first, you might have a tendency to list many weaknesses and scarcely any good points at all. But go back to the list every day and you'll eventually see all those wonderful, unsuspected qualities you've been hiding from yourself.

Being creative is another effective approach: paint, sing or sculpt without thinking about the result; just focus on the pleasure the act itself is giving you. Once again, you'll surprise yourself. Gardening and cooking may be thought of as less artistic but they are more practical ways of allowing your creative side to express itself.

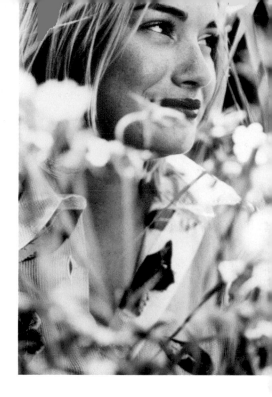

KEY FACTS

* Skin problems are exacerbated by a lack of self-confidence.

* To gain confidence, try using some personal-development methods, such as listing your good points or being creative.

* If that doesn't work, try psychotherapy.

60 calm down!

You get annoyed and your face starts to burn. You have an argument and your skin gets covered in blotches. Control your temper and never look like a beetroot again.

Anger and nettle rash As anyone will tell you, anger makes your cheeks go red. This is one of several physiological phenomena that enable our skin to reveal our emotions, most especially anger. Dermatologists interested in the relationship between the mind and the body also are aware that repressed anger can cause severe outbreaks of nettle rash.

Express yourself, but don't explode If you are prone to allergic nettle rash, it is likely that your skin will react in a similar way when you let your emotions get out of control. The solution sounds simple, but is not so easy to put into practice: learn to express what you feel calmly; don't lose your temper but don't suppress what you are feeling, either.

● ● ● DID YOU KNOW?

> To express yourself calmly, concentrate on what you want to say, not on what the other person is saying.
> Repeat yourself as often as you like, but never shout.
> Lower your voice. The other person will have to concentrate to hear your words, and their temper will subside. Suddenly you will both be having a civilized discussion.

KEY FACTS

* Suppressed emotions reveal themselves on your skin. Repressed anger, for example, can provoke nettle rash.

* Learn to express what you are feeling without losing your temper.

case study

I've finally accepted myself as I am

« Don't talk to me about eczema! I was covered with it for twenty years. At first, it was obviously an allergy: face creams, make-up and perfumes all caused reactions. I also reacted to some foods, particularly peanuts, almonds and walnuts. I made the best of it and accepted it as a fact of life. The blotches came and went. But they really took hold when my first serious relationship ended. I looked horrible! I didn't dare go out and just hid myself away. I looked as ugly as I felt and generally hated myself. I didn't make the link, of course. But a doctor helped me put my finger on it. I began to think about myself, my allergic reactions, the events of my life and I noticed some links, some strange coincidences. I took a few courses that taught me to accept myself and express myself. They were a great help. Ever since I started to accept myself as I am, I've benefited in two ways: I'm much happier and my eczema has cleared up completely. »

useful addresses

» Acupuncture

British Acupuncture Council
63 Jeddo Road
London W12 9HQ
tel: 020 8735 0400
www.acupuncture.org.uk

**British Medical
Acupuncture Society**
12 Marbury House
Higher Whitley, Warrington
Cheshire WA4 4QW.
tel: 01925 730727

**Australian Acupuncture
and Chinese Medicine Assn**
PO Box 5142, West End
Queensland 4101
Australia
www.acupuncture.org.au

» Allergies

Action Against Allergy
PO Box 278
Twickenham TW1 4QQ
tel: 020 8892 2711
www.actionagainstallergy.co.uk

British Allergy Foundation
Deepdene House
30 Bellegrove Rd, Welling
Kent DA16 3PY
tel: 0208 303 8525
www.allergyfoundation.com

**The Food Allergy and
Anaphylaxis Network**
11781 Lee Jackson Hwy
Suite 160, Fairfax
VA 22033-3309, USA
tel: 800-929-4040
www.foodallergy.org

**American Academy
of Allergy, Asthma and
Immunology**
611 East Wells St
Milwaukee, WI 53202
tel: (414) 272-6071
www.aaaai.org

» Herbal medicine

**British Herbal Medicine
Association**
Sun House, Church Street
Stroud, Gloucester GL5 1JL
tel: 01453 751389

**National Institute
of Medical Herbalists**
56 Longbrook Street
Exeter, Devon EX4 6AH
tel: 01392 426022

» Homeopathy

British Homeopathic Assn
Hahnemann House
29 Park Street West
Luton LU1 3BE
tel: 0870 444 3950

The Society of Homeopaths
4a Artizan Road
Northampton NN1 4HU
tel: 01604 621400

**Australian Homeopathic
Association**
PO Box 430, Hastings
Victoria 3915
Australia
www.homeopathyoz.org

» Relaxation therapy

British Autogenic Society
The Royal London
Homoeopathic Hospital
Greenwell Street
London W1W 5BP
www.autogenic-therapy.org.uk

**British Complementary
Medicine Association**
PO Box 5122
Bournemouth BH8 0WG
tel: 0845 345 5977
www.bcma.co.uk

» Yoga

The British Wheel of Yoga
25 Jermyn Street
Sleaford
Lincs NG34 7RU
tel: 01529 306 851
www.bwy.org.uk

index

acknowledgements

Cover: B. Bailey/Getty Images: p.8-9: Neo Vision/Photonica; p.10: Neo Vision/Photonica; p.12: Neo Vision/Photonica; p.14: M. Barraud/Getty Images; p.16: Neo Vision/Photonica; p.20: S.Watson/Getty Images; p.22: A. Nagelmann/Getty Images; p.24: S. Simpson/Getty Images; p.27: Neo Vision/Photonica; p.29: T. Garcia/Getty Images; p.31: C. Harvey/Getty Images; p.35: Johner/Photonica; p.36: T. Reed/Zefa; p.39: Neo Vision/Photonica; p.40: Akiko Ida; p.45: Neo Vision/Photonica; p.48-49: A. Miksch/Getty Images; p.51: J. Lamb/Getty Images; p.53: J.Toy/Getty Images; p.54-55: M. Cashew/ Photonica; p.57: F.Tousche/Getty Images; p.58: P.Nicholson/Getty Images; p.60: H. Benser/Zefa; p.62: G. Buss/Getty Images; p.69:T. Krüsselmann/Zefa; p.71: A. Lichtenberg/Getty Images; p.72: R. Daly/Getty Images; p.79: K. Lili/Zefa; p.81: J. Darell/Getty Images; p.86-87: VCL/Getty Images; p.89: P.Nicholson/Getty Images; p.90, 92: Akiko Ida; p.95: S. Ragland/Getty Images; p.100: Photodisc; p.103: Emely/Zefa; p.104: Neo Vision/Photonica; p.107: S. Casimiro/Getty Images; p.108: K. Mikami/Photonica; p.113: J. Franco/Getty Images; p.114: /Option Photo; p.121: P. Beavis/Zefa.

Ilustrations: Philippe Doro pages 42, 82 and 96; Hélène Lafaix pages 66-67, 76-77 and 116-117; Anne Cinquanta pages 118-119.

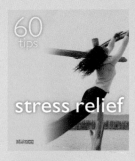

stress relief

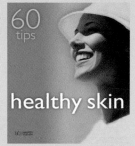

healthy skin

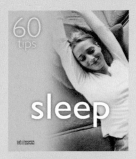

sleep

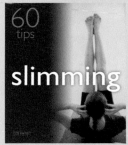

slimming

The 60 Tips
collection
All the keys,
all the tips
and all the
answers to
your health
questions

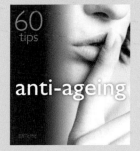

anti-ageing

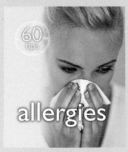

allergies

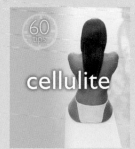

cellulite

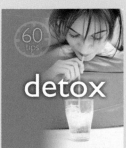

detox

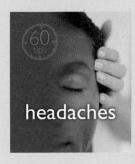

headaches

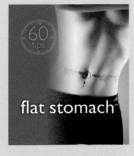

flat stomach

Series editor: Marie Borrel

Editorial directors: Delphine Kopff and Caroline Rolland

Editorial assistants: Delphine Kopff and Anne Vallet

Graphic design and layout: G & C MOI

Preparation, final checking: Chloé Chauveau and Aurélie Pugeaut

Illustrations: Guylaine Moi

Production: Felicity O'Connor

Colour separations: IGS-Charente photogravure Angoulême

Translation: JMS Books LLP

© Hachette Livre (Hachette Pratique) 2003
This edition published in 2004 by Hachette Illustrated UK, Octopus Publishing Group Ltd.,
2–4 Heron Quays, London E14 4JP

English translation by JMS Books LLP (email: moseleystrachan@blueyonder.co.uk)
Translation © Octopus Publishing Group Ltd.

A CIP catalogue for this book is available from the British Library

ISBN-13: 978-1-84430-093-8

ISBN-10: 1-84430-093-5

Printed in Singapore by Tien Wah Press